Advance Praise for
Optimizing Your Health

"In this lucidly written book, Emily Gold Mears provides a roadmap for individuals to understand their own bodies and enact different behaviors and regimens to achieve good health and wellness. She does not use jargon or patronize the reader but rather explains concepts clearly and succinctly while pointing to additional resources, including clinical trials and reputable research studies. The penultimate chapter on using to evidence to understand science and medicine is especially helpful in elucidating the potential as well as limitations of different types of clinical investigation. If only all people were as proactive, data-driven, rigorous, and scientifically curious as Gold Mears! With this book, she gives readers an opportunity to be so and to work (it definitely takes work, as she shows!) toward greater health."

— AARON F. MERTZ, Ph.D.,
Director, Aspen Institute
Science & Society Program

"Emily Gold Mears offers the public an extraordinary gift. The current pandemic has reminded us all in graphic and compelling ways that we have ultimate responsibility for our own health. For best outcomes with our medical professional partners, we must nonetheless navigate enormous amounts of information from seemingly infinite origins, often contradictory and confusing. As a citizen scientist and unbiased advocate for responsible, effective, evidenced-based healthcare, Ms. Gold Mears provides a framework for us to make the most well-informed medical decisions. She translates primary source cutting-edge clinical research into clear protocols for action. As a psychiatrist focusing on epigenetics and brain health, I hope every patient with whom I consult will utilize this excellent comprehensive resource. They would be able to engage in more meaningful dialogue and ask better questions to the desired end of truly optimizing their health and well-being. I further hope the public more generally will do the same, ultimately elevating the common good."

— RONNIE S. STANGLER, M.D.,
Clinical Professor Emerita, University of Washington, Department of Psychiatry and Behavioral Sciences, Founder, Genome Advisory

"Emily Gold Mears has written a truly approachable guide that seeks to make sense out of the torrent of sometime contradictory novel information that is emerging around age-old topics like diet, exercise, and sleep while exploring cutting-edge research and its health implications in areas like the genome and the microbiome. Throughout, she brings a distinctive voice filled with curiosity and humility, leavened by personal stories that humanize the science she is summarizing and that illuminate the fundamental human desire to help us all live longer, healthier, and happier lives."

— ROBERT C. GREEN, M.D., M.P.H.,
Professor of Medicine (Genetics), Director, Genomes2People Research Program/Preventive Genomics Clinic/Population Precision Health at Ariadne Labs, Mass General Brigham, Broad Institute, Ariadne Labs, Harvard Medical School

OPTIMIZING YOUR HEALTH

AN **APPROACHABLE** GUIDE
TO **REDUCING** YOUR RISK
OF **CHRONIC** DISEASE

EMILY GOLD MEARS

Post Hill
PRESS

A POST HILL PRESS BOOK
ISBN: 978-1-63758-291-6
ISBN (eBook): 978-1-63758-292-3

Optimizing Your Health:
An Approachable Guide to Reducing Your Risk of Chronic Disease
© 2022 by Emily Gold Mears
All Rights Reserved

Post Hill Press
New York • Nashville
posthillpress.com

Published in the United States of America

1 2 3 4 5 6 7 8 9 10

*To my father who was brilliant, funny, and
had an unwavering sense of morality.
I miss him every day.*

TABLE OF CONTENTS

FOREWORD

by William P. Stanford, MD, PhD, FACP

I FIRST MET EMILY AT an A4M meeting in Las Vegas in December of 2019. As a physician-scientist and Chief Medical/Scientific Officer of the Beverly Hills Institute for Precision Medicine (BHIPM), I was attending the conference to learn more about integrative medicine. My primary interest in personalized precision medicine demands a clinical literacy in integrative medicine, as there is much overlap between the two fields of integrative and precision medicine.

Emily was sitting a few rows away from me toward the front and center of the audience. One could not help but notice the rapt attention that she gave to the speaker alongside her furious scribbling of notes. She asked a very intelligent and relevant question of the speaker who was quite bullish and aggressive in their self-promotion of a controversial, poorly scientifically supported position on a widely controversial treatment for anti-aging. It was clear that Emily was neither intimidated nor outgunned as she made her inquiry. I made a note to self: get to know this physician or scientist before the end of the conference.

I followed Emily out of the hotel ballroom; another attendee had in mind my same agenda, and stopped her in the broad expanse of a hallway. As I approached, the other attendee was complimenting her on her line of questioning and iterating the notion of their struggle and shyness to pursue a similar line of questioning. I piped in my admiration for the question as well. I introduced myself and asked her name and where she practiced. I was very surprised at the response. She stated that she was neither a physician nor a scientist; in fact, her education was in law. She attended conferences such as these in search of new promising therapies to potentially avail herself to inform friends and colleagues. She also mentioned that she was on the lookout for smart, talented healthcare providers that she could engage in her own care, as well as companies that may be investable.

I was thrilled to learn Emily lived in the Los Angeles area like me and we arranged a meeting to discuss her thoughts on the future of medicine from the "consumer" standpoint and the vast library of information that she had accumulated in her efforts to inform her own health plan. I quickly realized that this perspective from such an intelligent and informed consumer of avant-garde science would be a huge asset to those of us working in translational medicine as we attempt to bring bona fide medical breakthroughs from the lab to the clinic.

Though this gold mine of a "focus group of one" was a bonanza for my team's enterprise efforts at BHIPM, it was also easy to see that Emily possessed a great fund of knowledge that would benefit her fellow like-minded proactive healthcare purveyors. Emily related how she had begun a blog with a focus on dementia—the disease that devastated her beloved father. I visited the blog site and was very impressed again with her knowledge and her writing skill. The "Captain Obvious" in me asked Emily if she had ever considered writing a book and sharing her expanse of hard-earned medical intelligence with the public. She said that the idea had crossed her mind, though the sheer volume of notes, memos, and medical records made the prospect of organizing all of it into a manuscript somewhat prohibitive.

I encouraged (okay, begged) her to do so, as I felt that her experience and effort in acquiring and cataloguing this information would be of huge benefit to all patients and the vast number of consumers who are entering the precision health and wellness marketplace.

Fortunately for us, Emily made this effort, working many months on the manuscript. She has produced a magnificently well organized, thoughtful treatise on how a healthcare consumer can approach this mystery of futuristic precision medicine and help themselves to optimal health and longevity. Congratulations, Emily, and thank you for writing this book.

WHY THIS BOOK:
You Must Become Your Own Health Advocate

THE UNITED STATES IS BECOMING the sickest nation in the Western world because of the epidemic of chronic disease. According to the CDC, 60 percent of American adults have a chronic disease and 40 percent have two or more, and these numbers are growing. More than half of Americans rely on daily doses of pharmaceuticals. One hundred years ago, the most common cause of death was infection. Now, chronic degenerative disease represents the number one global health threat. Disease is defined as "impaired normal functioning" and represents a collection of symptoms.

In fact, most of these diseases such as metabolic syndrome, obesity, type 2 diabetes, cardiovascular disease, neurodegenerative disease, and even some cancers, can be prevented by altering lifestyle choices.

This book is written for anyone who wants to lower their risk of getting a chronic disease and for anyone interested in learning about the many lifestyle adjustments that can help optimize your health and resilience. This book will offer smart strategies and tips as well as explanations and resources for health optimization. It will illustrate where conventional medicine is helpful and when you should consider functional medicine as an alternative approach. More than ever before, each of us must take control of our own health and become as resilient as we can to withstand the ubiquitous health challenges that we face.

I wrote this book as a mother of two sons, a daughter of a father who died from a chronic disease, and as a patient myself. After a lifetime of disregarding all aspects of my health, I have altered my lifestyle in pursuit of optimal health and resilience. I want to share what I have learned so others can feel great and lower their chronic disease risk.

> As a lawyer, a citizen scientist, and a health and science advocate, I took every possible measure to check and verify my sources.

I primarily relied upon clinical studies and papers published in highly regarded scientific and medical publications. The absolute glut of pseudoscience and misinformation is a serious problem. People are confused and misguided. There needs to be a trustworthy source that disseminates actionable and accurate information. That is why I have written this book.

I have focused on eighteen different areas to consider when altering your lifestyle. Due to the lack of potential profit, the business community lacks the financial incentive to promote these simple methods of health optimization. Each chapter will include at least five actionable steps succinctly illustrated to begin the critical adjustments. There will be a resource section at the back of the book to list the most reliable and trustworthy brands. I have no affiliation whatsoever with any of the companies, products, brands, or services listed in the resource section. I offer these merely as suggestions. For the most part, the book is based on the new branch of medicine that has emerged to deal with the diseases that conventional medicine is not designed to treat. This area of medicine is called functional medicine. The relatively new disciplines of integrative and personalized medicine will also be helpful in the treatment of chronic diseases. Functional medicine is an approach that attempts to identify the root cause of disease. Critics claim that this area of medicine is not evidence-based and is not supported by research. That is a baseless criticism and is largely because the studies are harder to search for and locate online. PubMed is a database where studies on life sciences and biomedical topics can be found, and there needs to be a similar site for functional medicine studies.

The "medical-industrial complex" manages conventional medicine based upon the management of symptoms with medications or surgery. It treats disease from a linear, singular cause-and-effect model that may not take the body as a whole into account. This area of medicine focuses on the diagnosis of disease and symptom treatment. It doesn't attempt to determine the root cause of a disease or symptom and often overlooks the consideration that we are all composed of biochemical, physiological, and genetic differences. Body systems are interconnected; altering just one thing does not work.

> Each chapter and different topic will have at least five actionable steps succinctly illustrated to begin the critical adjustments.

This book will show you how to avoid chronic disease by making changes that respond to the multiple factors contributing to these diseases. These differences are significant because they account for our varied responses to, well, just about everything. In no way am I disparaging conventional medical care with a broad brushstroke. I am quick to give credit for improvements in anesthesia, blood transfusion, antibiotics, and the handling of acute care situations. But our severely flawed health-care system is designed to treat diseases, not prevent them. Many health issues can be improved or eliminated by certain lifestyle modifications. I am not suggesting that it is easy to make these modifications, but making them is essential to your optimal health.

Behavior is one of the most difficult things to change, and this is illustrated by the vast number of books written about how to change one's behavior.

> There is a prominent place for both health officials and the government to improve societal health, but ultimately, it is up to each one of us to take our individual health into our own hands.

We have to find a way to encourage people to value and prioritize health over all else, and the government will need to step in and subsidize this effort. Most people are aware that good nutrition, exercise, sleep, and the avoidance of tobacco and excessive alcohol lead to good health. I realize that there is an argument as to whether these represent "choices" to many. The lack of access for many in our society to healthy food choices and air and water quality and exposure to environmental toxins is a monumental problem that must be addressed. This crisis is an area where the government will have to step in and provide assistance. It will be necessary for experts across many fields to help frame policy to promote societal health.

I suspect another issue is that many people believe that it is too hard to be healthy with all of the temptations. Behavioral science reveals that people resist doing something inconsistent with their beliefs. This same field suggests that if people change their thoughts, their behavior will follow. In other words, if people could be persuaded to believe that they absolutely could be healthy, the requisite behavior will follow. Procrastination about getting healthy is also ubiquitous. I think this is because chronic diseases progress very slowly and are often asymptomatic at the onset. Due to evolutionary reasons, we tend to respond to that which is immediately in front of us and rarely exercise any long-range foresight.

In most cases, the body is designed brilliantly. We have a natural ability to heal. If we had not developed excellent immunity, we would have died out as a race thousands of years ago. As environmental factors enter to disrupt the natural balance, we must support our bodies' natural biological process of repair and function. Our bodies are made up of complex interconnected systems. We should think of our bodies as human operating systems and employ a systems-engineering approach. NASA defines this approach as a "methodical, disciplined approach for the design, realization, technical management, and operations of a system."

Unfortunately, the health-care industry profits from sick people. The industry did not devise health care to help patients avoid illness. We must redesign the system to prioritize prevention over profit. While humans tend to ignore long-term planning, the reality is that improvements in a population's health can and will lead to reductions in health costs. I don't love the term prevention because I don't think it's realistic to "prevent" every eventuality. I will use the term prevention going forward because it has already received attention. I would prefer an emphasis on building individual *resilience*. If you could become as resilient as possible, you would need not be concerned with what unpreventable forces are out there.

The other issue I have with prevention is that it is difficult to measure. I believe that you can't improve what you can't measure, and it is possible to measure certain metrics of resilience. There

Think of our body's systems as a bucket. As toxins and morbidities drip into the bucket, our system can handle them—until a point when the bucket fills and the contents spill out. By adopting behaviors that reduce stress, toxins, and damage to our systems, we reduce the water level in the bucket.

have been many attempts at "prevention" in the past, but I believe that most are based upon faulty science. They include putting lead and fluoride in the water, folic acid and synthetic vitamins in the food supply, and vaccinations. Vaccinations are responsible for eradicating many horrible diseases and have improved the quality of life for the global population. We have new viral threats spurred by the effects of globalization and climate change. Vaccinations cannot be the only mode of prevention as we advance in human history.

The extreme variable responses to COVID-19 illustrate the need for public health initiatives to focus on prevention beyond vaccines. Public health will become more precise as emerging technology and data tools become more widely available. When this occurs, we can leave behind the ineffective one-size-fits-all protocol that defines and dehumanizes medicine today. We are each unique in our response to everything and should not all be treated the same.

Along with functional, integrative, and precision medicine, the growing field of "wellness" has emerged to address issues that conventional medicine has failed to address. In fact, wellness is a mostly unregulated industry valued at $4.2 trillion. I think the name is rather flimsy and not sufficiently descriptive. The industry has fostered unregulated practices, inadequate training, and expensive tests. There needs to be an effective way to distinguish between pseudoscientific claims and those with legitimate approaches. Perhaps the future will require that claims and brands need to be certified by a regulatory body to save consumers from the unscrupulous ones. In the meanwhile, there are efforts toward vetting some.

Note the Instagram account, Estée Laundry. It goes after false claims from "influencers" and bad brands in the beauty industry. CVS has an initiative called "Tested to Be Trusted" which subjects all of its vitamins and supplements to third-party testing. Senator Richard Blumenthal of Connecticut inquired into Rite Aid's "Wellness Ambassadors" to uncover deceptive and misleading practices at the chain. There is a website called www.wellnessevidence.com that investigates the accuracy, safety, and efficacy of wellness claims.

There needs to be an effort to educate consumers on how to distinguish between fact and fiction and between science and marketing.

I based my research on voraciously reading books on different health topics, attending scientific, medical, and biohacking conferences, taking online classes, occupying seats on scientific and medical-related boards, and extensively researching PubMed, Google Scholar, and other scientific databases containing peer-reviewed studies.

Through my extensive research, I have found information that has been largely limited to the scientific community. Some of this information challenges our preconceived notions and suggests new approaches. But all of it is actionable and can help us not only reduce our risk for chronic disease but also mitigate the debilitating consequences of chronic disease.

> People need to know that they can and must take ownership of their health, and that if they do, they will have the opportunity to feel better, live longer, and postpone the onset and mitigate the consequences of chronic disease.

The approach to health care and the lifestyle alterations about which I write can make a significant difference in the health of our nation.

CHAPTER 1

YOUR ORAL MICROBIOME:
The First Line of Defense

MY FRIEND STEVEN WAS ALWAYS talking about his sensitive teeth. If he ate or drank anything too hot, too cold, or too crunchy he felt pain in his teeth and mouth. He had visited dentist after dentist, all of whom simply recommended that he switch to a toothpaste for "sensitive teeth." He tried doing that until I asked him to look at the ingredients in those toothpastes. He learned that the ingredients included potassium nitrate, stannous fluoride, sodium saccharin, Blue 1, sorbitol, pentasodium triphosphate, PEG-8, SLS, xanthan gum, sodium hydroxide, and cocamidopropyl betaine. Other than the initial conclusion that these are not substances that occur in nature, most of us have no understanding of these ingredients. Steven decided that the last thing he wanted to do was to add chemicals to his already sensitive teeth.

A few of the dentists who Steven visited pointed out that he had accumulated an excessive amount of plaque. In dentist speak, plaque is a sticky biofilm that develops when bacteria collects where the teeth meet the gumline. Biofilms are not always bad. They can be protective or harmful, depending on the type of bacteria forming to create them. Everyone has biofilms. Problems arise when you have too many or they are formed by pathogenic bacteria which cause your gums to become inflamed and bleed.

The third oral issue that plagued Steven was persistent bad breath, or halitosis. Steven learned that bad breath has many causes including eating certain foods, poor dental hygiene, and inflammation. His bad breath was related to his gum disease. I suggested that Steven prioritize his oral health because while sensitive teeth, plaque, and bad breath are annoying and unpleasant, if left untreated, these issues can lead to cardiovascular disease, Alzheimer's disease, diabetes, obesity, digestive disorders, rheumatoid arthritis, and even infertility.

Steven found a holistic/biological dentist who used a different approach than the other dentists he had seen. His new dentist investigated the imbalances in his mouth to determine the cause of his sensitive teeth, excessive biofilms, and bad breath. Some of the steps that Steven added to his oral hygiene routine included tongue scraping, careful flossing, use of a nontoxic toothpaste, the elimination of an alcohol-based mouthwash, and an oral probiotic designed specifically for oral health.

Optimal health begins in your mouth.

According to Donna E. Shalala, former Secretary of Health and Human Services, "Oral health means more than healthy teeth and you cannot be healthy without oral health."[1] The word *oral* is defined as including not only the teeth, gums, and supporting tissue, but also the hard and soft palate, the mucosal lining of the mouth and throat, the tongue, the lips, the salivary glands, the chewing muscles, and the jaw.

> Your mouth is the gateway to your digestive health. While the gut is central to human health, the health of the gut is directly influenced by oral health. There is a clear bidirectional relationship between our oral health and our systemic wellness.

MICROBES IN YOUR MOUTH

Second only to the gut, the mouth is filled with a large and diverse selection of microbes. These microorganisms take up residence on the teeth, tongue, cheeks, gums, tonsils, and palate. Both the normal temperature of one's mouth, the range of which is 36.1–37.5°C (97–99.6°F) as well as the stable pH of saliva, the normal range of which is 6.2–7.6, make for an ideal environment for the microbes. It makes sense that the oral cavity is the first point of entry to the digestive and respiratory tract. Every time you swallow, you are sending bacteria, fungi, Protozoa, and viruses from your mouth down into your gastrointestinal tract. This impacts your immune system. Holistic dentist Steven Lin, DDS, writes in his book *The Dental Diet*, "We swallow trillions of bacteria every day. That's thousands a second. If that isn't a profound marker of how important your mouth is, then it's hard to see what possibly could be! One of the biggest advances in medicine in recent years is the appreciation of the gut microbiome and its role in chronic diseases all over the body. The mouth is unequivocally linked to your gut, so your oral microbiome is a measurable and accessible way to see how your body is working." Bacteria have many different functions. The good ones transport minerals from saliva to the teeth and aid in the mineralization of teeth. Other bacteria carry oxygen to the gums and soft tissues. This aids in the excretion of waste and prevents disease-causing microbes from causing infection.

DIGESTION BEGINS IN YOUR MOUTH

We cannot ignore the fact that digestion begins in the mouth and that chewing prompts saliva production. A lack of sufficient saliva translates to a dry mouth. When your salivary flow is reduced, so is the secretion of digestive proteins that begin the digestive process. When the mouth is overly dry, bacterial overgrowth is encouraged which leads to cavities, gum disease, and bad breath. Some of the causes of dry mouth include underlying disease, dehydration, some pharmaceuticals, tobacco and alcohol use, and snoring or sleeping with your mouth open. The technical name for dry mouth is xerostomia.

European dentists have acknowledged the connection between the oral cavity and overall health. In the US, the medical and dental professions work independently of each other and neglect to accept the interdependence of the two disciplines. Conventional dentists in the US tend to be concerned only with the treatment of misaligned teeth, cavities, and gum disease. Unless they have studied to become a holistic dentist, most dentists are not concerned with the relationship between the oral microbiome and GI tract disorders, the immune system, heart health, gut-brain axis, and endocrine system disorders.

CHRONIC INFLAMMATION LEADS TO DISEASE

In the words of Dr. Barry Sears, "silent inflammation is a condition that occurs when the body's natural immune response goes awry." It is linked to a long list of health threats and can continue for years undetected. There is an important distinction between acute inflammation and chronic inflammation, which I will describe in detail in chapter 3. For now, it's important to note that while acute inflammation is a vital process that contributes to healing, chronic inflammation is the precursor to disease. The detection of inflammation in your mouth is as critical to treatment as it is for the rest of your body. Poisons in the mouth can threaten one's optimal immune system. The list of contributors to chronic inflammation is quite long. It includes bleeding gums, gingivitis, periodontal disease, infected teeth, cavitations, and failed root canals just to begin. Other contributors will be discussed in the chapter on inflammation.

BEWARE OF GUM DISEASE

Gingivitis is defined as inflammation of the outermost soft tissue of the gums, or gingiva.[2] The gingiva becomes red and prone to bleeding and is usually caused by a bacterial infection. If left untreated, it can progress to periodontitis.

Periodontitis is a serious gum infection that can damage both the soft tissue as well as the jawbone supporting the teeth. The hallmark of this condition is a biofilm (defined as a thin, slimy film of bacteria that adheres to a surface) causing bacterial endotoxins to cause pockets between the gum and the teeth.[3] Bacteria grow in the pockets and the bone structure becomes damaged. Not only does this condition have a severely adverse effect on one's oral cavity, but it is also a serious risk factor for diabetes, cardiovascular, pulmonary, and neurological disease.[4] "The oral microbiome rests within biofilms throughout the oral cavity and forms an ecosystem that maintains health in a state of equilibrium. When this equilibrium is disrupted, dysbiosis occurs and pathogens enter and contribute to disease."[5]

It is a good rule of thumb to remember that in medicine, anything ending in "itis" indicates inflammation and usually is the suffix used to describe an inflammatory disease.

A study conducted by the CDC reveals that nearly half of Americans over the age of thirty and over 70 percent of those aged sixty-five or over have periodontal disease.[6,7]

The excessive growth of these disease-causing organisms contributes to disorders of the brain, heart, lungs, kidney, liver, bone, vascular system, nervous system, endocrine system, and a general reduction of optimal immune functioning.

> The impact of poor oral health is vast and affects the entire body. When one neglects proper care of their mouth, pathogenic organisms are free to grow out of control.

CAVITIES ARE A RED FLAG FOR BIGGER ISSUES

Tooth decay is a result of poor oral health and a contributor to chronic inflammation and disease. For years, scientists have not been able to definitively identify the cause of tooth decay. There have been several theories including the degree of enamel hardness and bacterial plaque forming on teeth because of consuming acidic or sugary foods or drinks. Ralph Steinman, a dentist at the University of Loma Linda who studied the dentinal fluid transport system was among the first to conclude that tooth decay is a systemic health issue. His research published in 1958 stated that sugar intake, stress, certain pharmaceuticals, lack of exercise, and a lack of micronutrients all influence this dentinal fluid transport system. While his work is old, it still stands today as the explanation for how our teeth have built-in defensive responses to protect us. Everything we consume, including food, drinks, pharmaceuticals, and toxins, affects our blood chemistry. Our brain responds to the state of our blood chemistry by sending a message to the parotid gland (the largest salivary gland, located in the front and just below the ears) which then communicates with your teeth. The result of this salivary-led communication is to remineralize your teeth, which causes them to be stronger. If your teeth are stronger, they will have greater success in resisting bacteria.

Each tooth is a living organism with its own nerve and blood supply. Tooth decay or cavities, as we call them, are referred to as dental caries. It is widely accepted that tooth decay is linked to nutrition—specifically our industrialized diets. Dr. Weston Price studied the diets of Aboriginal tribes to test his dental hypotheses. He found that prior to introducing modern foods into their diets, the Aboriginal tribes lived for generations without cavities. Their diet contained no sugar, grains, legumes, or nuts and they were immune to tooth decay. Grains, legumes, and nuts present an issue because they contain phytic acid which inhibits the absorption of vitamins and minerals in the digestive tract. Dr. Price is known to have declared that "tooth decay is not only unnecessary, but an indication of our divergence from nature's fundamental laws of life and health."

I must point out that Dr. Weston Price is the subject of a great deal of criticism and has been accused of promoting theories that are not based on scientific evidence. While his research may have been somewhat flawed, I believe that his connection between diet and oral health is correct. He lived and conducted his studies during the latter part of the twentieth century and the early twenty-first century, and simply because his work does not exactly conform to conventional dentistry, he is criticized. This exemplifies a big problem today. Anything that does not reflect conventional medicine or dentistry or is not the subject of randomized placebo-controlled studies is passed off as "alternative" and quackery. I believe this is shortsighted. While I am sensitive to the issue of pseudoscience, just because something may have been discovered without a gold-standard study does not in and of itself invalidate the discovery. There are many occasions when observational studies are accurate. For instance, one does not need to run a randomized, placebo-controlled study to know for certain that the likelihood of fire is increased when leaving matches with a group of small children. I am unaware of anyone or any clinical study that has disproved Dr. Price's link between diet and tooth decay. As a matter of fact, a chapter of the book *Microbiology of Dental Decay and Periodontal Disease* by W. J. Loesche identifies that dental decay became an important health problem when sucrose became a major component of the human diet.[8] The book goes on to point out that "when sucrose is consumed frequently, an organism known as *Streptococcus mutans* emerges as the predominant organism, and it is this organism that has been uniquely associated with dental decay." Later studies suggest that the presence of *Streptococcus mutans* may, in fact, be the result of tooth decay, not the cause of it.[9] It is suggested in the book *Holistic Dental Care* by Stephen A. Lawrence that cavities are not due to sugar and bacteria on your teeth, but rather they are due to an imbalance in the body's hypothalamus gland.

SILVER AMALGAMS

As controversial as the work of Dr. Weston Price is, the controversy surrounding silver amalgams is huge. To begin this discussion, one must at least consider the premise that many believe that current dental practices are quite primitive. When one gets a cavity, which is essentially a small hole in the tooth, the dentist then drills a bigger hole in the same tooth and fills that hole with synthetic material. Most of the synthetic materials are toxic and some (though not all) people experience an adverse effect from them. While the adverse effect is usually subtle and gradually degrades the immune system, the entire process renders the tooth weak and traumatized and usually results in the need for a crown or a root canal years later. As of September 24, 2020, the FDA issued recommendations about dental amalgams in certain groups who may be at greater risk of the potential adverse health effects of mercury exposure. While the FDA stops short of recommending the removal of existing silver amalgams or banning any use of these mercury-filled deposits in one's mouth, they do list the potential adverse health effects of mercury exposure from dental amalgams. This strikes me as hypocritical. The FDA acknowledges that mercury exposure through dental amalgams can be harmful but limits that harm to only certain individuals "at greater risk." I cannot help but wonder, who is mercury exposure, a known neurotoxin, good for? The American Dental Association currently claims that silver amalgams are safe, long lasting, economical, and inert. While it is true that they are relatively inexpensive and they do last many years, the science supports the claim that they are not inert and mercury vapor is released.[10],[11] While the status may be considered "not definitive" and, perhaps, could depend upon the underlying health and genetics of the individual patient, the dental schools and the profession are changing, and about 50 percent fewer dentists still place silver amalgams. Mark C. Houston, a cardiovascular disease specialist, states that "the overall vascular effects of mercury include increased oxidative stress and inflammation, reduced oxidative defense, thrombosis, vascular smooth muscle dysfunction, endothelial dysfunction, dyslipidemia, and immune and mitochondrial dysfunction."[12] He goes on to say that "the clinical consequences of mercury toxicity include hypertension, coronary heart disease, myocardial infarction, cardiac arrhythmias, reduced heart rate variability, increased carotid intima-media thickness and carotid artery obstruction, cerebrovascular accident, generalized atherosclerosis, and renal dysfunction." Brushing teeth, chewing food, grinding the teeth, and consuming very acidic foods and carbonated sodas all contribute to the outgassing of mercury.

ROOT CANALS

Another subject of great controversy is that of root canal–treated teeth. The main governing body of endodontists (dentists who perform root canals) claims that root canals are a safe and effective procedure. There is an enormous body of literature based on research that confirms that root canal–treated teeth remain infected and that 40 percent of these teeth have been proven to have chronic apical periodontitis (CAP), which is the most severe periodontal disease.

There is a fascinating book, *Hidden Epidemic: Silent Oral Infections Cause Most Heart Attacks and Breast Cancers*, written by Dr. Thomas Levy. He is a board-certified cardiologist who extensively researched the connection between dental work and toxicity. He focused on "silent oral infections," those which are frequently painless, and listed several serious illnesses that have been linked to these infections. His book lists several different types of cancers,

Alzheimer's disease, Parkinson's disease, diabetes, hypertension, lupus, arthritis, and other diseases as being linked to oral infections and the resulting inflammation. Despite decades of people insisting that there is no scientific link between root canal–treated teeth and chronic disease, the current peer-reviewed studies suggest otherwise.[13],[14] Personally, I had one root canal–treated tooth. In my attempt to achieve optimal health, I had it removed. I did not do this impulsively, but rather I did so after extensive research. I had to first find the appropriate dental professional for the job, and I had what is called a 3D cone beam imaging X-ray to reveal the underlying infection. A conventional dental X-ray does not have the ability to reveal possible, underlying infections.

FLUORIDE

Yet one more topic of controversy is fluoride. While most conventional dentists recommend the use of toothpastes containing fluoride and insist that it is safe, the reality is that fluoride is only safe, if at all, at extremely low concentrations. At high doses, ingestion of fluoride is lethal. The CDC and the American Dental Association warn about the dangers of swallowing more than an amount the size of one rice grain worth of fluoride containing toothpaste. An article states that "tooth decay is not caused by fluoride deficiency [...] and fluoride supplementation can't reverse active cavities."[15] I am neither a dental nor a medical professional and I do not want to advise you, but I would certainly take this information under consideration.

ORAL CARE AND GERIATRICS

The impact of the health of one's oral activity has enormous relevance in geriatric care. It is suggested in studies that tooth loss may be a risk factor for the decline of cognitive functions. Several stud-

ies have been conducted about the interaction between mastica-
tion and cognition.[16] While studies have not been conclusive, it has
been found that patients in nursing homes with the highest rate of
dementia had the fewest teeth.

In January 2020, Debora Mackenzie wrote in *New Scientist* about
the theory that Alzheimer's disease could be caused in part by a
bacterial infection.[17] The article discusses the gum-disease-causing
organism called *Porphyromonas gingivalis* and its adverse effect on
one's immune system. This bacterium causes inflammation and can
be difficult to treat. Other studies have confirmed that *P. gingivalis*
has been found in the hippocampus, the memory center of the brain
in Alzheimer's patients.[18]

MY STORY

Personally, I have gone to great lengths to clean up my oral cavity.
My odyssey has included the removal of all of my silver amalgams
and my gold crowns. I felt strongly about having a metal-free mouth.
While gold is the least reactive metal of all of the metals used in dental materials, they are never composed of only gold. They are alloys,
which means that they contain other metals. It is possible that people who have strong immune systems can manage a mouth filled
with metal and that they don't wish to endure the expense and has-
sle of removal. My feeling is that we are exposed to so many toxins
everywhere that whatever one can do to reduce their exposure will be
beneficial. There is a relatively new test available called the MELISA
test, developed by Dr. Vera Stejskal. This is a blood test that will
reveal one's sensitivity and biocompatibility to not just dental material but also to those used for surgical implants and joint prostheses.
The website Melisa.org is a tremendous resource for relevant articles.

When I embarked on the odyssey of cleaning up my oral cavity,
I ended up at a dentist in New York City. This was not exactly conve-

nient since I live in Los Angeles, but I am delighted with my decision. As part of the regular exam, this dental office took a plaque sample from me and looked at it under a microscope. They did a salivary analysis to look for periodontal pathogens. This microscopic slide analysis has the potential of revealing bacteria, white blood cells, spirochetes, amoeba, and other opportunistic organisms. These organisms can indicate the presence of an infection that might otherwise remain undiscovered. Spirochetes are fascinating creatures and can live inside your body's cells and hide from your immune system. They can contribute to gum disease, heart disease, Alzheimer's disease, diabetes, autoimmune disease, and cancer. They can literally eat through the skin and drink blood and fibrin. It is thought that if your gums bleed easily, it is an indication of capillary fragility and the probable presence of spirochetes. I have read that despite the prevailing dental wisdom of flossing at least once a day, a Waterpik is a better tool for the removal of food in between one's teeth. This is because flossing can cause micro-ruptures in your gingiva and damage your gums.

In conclusion, the best approach to improving your oral microbiome is to employ the same principles to oral health as one should apply to their general health. Don't smoke, don't abuse alcohol or drugs, make sleep and exercise a priority, and above all, eat a nutrient-dense diet. Including taking vitamins A, B, C, D/K2, and even CoQ10 will help one's teeth fight off potential decay. I would also suggest staying away from certain chemicals that are ubiquitous in many dental products such as sodium lauryl sulfate and triclosan which can cause chronic oral irritation. While triclosan is banned for use in soap and other products because of its known risk to human health, it is still allowed to be used in toothpastes. Many whitening products contain potassium nitrate, which is something to avoid. Harmful chemicals from whitening strips and mouthwash strip your teeth of their protective layer. Mouthwash is used by many without the knowledge of its harmful effects. You should take note of the potential of mouthwash to alter your microbiome and damage teeth.[19] Scientists at the University of Plymouth have conducted studies on the long-term effects of chlorhexidine in mouthwash. They found that just one week of using mouthwash containing chlorhexidine can lower saliva pH, increase acidity, and increase the risk of tooth damage and reduce microbial diversity. Beneficial bacteria are reduced and harmful bacteria increased with the use of mouthwash containing this ingredient. There are several nontoxic brands available, but one must do continual research. Jāsön and Burt's Bees were two brands that had been trustworthy, but both have been purchased by Clorox and may have had ingredients changed. Tom's is another brand thought to be great, but it contains sodium lauryl sulfate. If you are interested in doing further research, I suggest that you consult the International Academy of Oral Medicine and Toxicology website: www.IAOMT.org.

The key to oral health is an ecologically balanced and diverse microbiome.

ACTION STEPS

➢ Consider your nutrition.

>   Too many refined carbohydrates cause tooth decay and
>   contribute to an imbalance of oral microbes. Add more
>   organic fruits and vegetables.

➢ Quit smoking.

➢ Stop using mouthwash, toothpaste, and other oral care products filled with chemicals.

>   These products are killing the good, necessary bacteria
>   along with the bad bacteria.

>   If the product contains alcohol, artificial sweeteners, coal
>   tar, color dyes, DEA (diethanolamine), microplastics, pro-
>   pylene glycol, sodium fluoride, sodium lauryl/laureth sul-
>   fate (SLS/SLE), or triclosan, do not use them!

➢ Make your oral hygiene a priority.

>   Brush, Floss, use a Waterpik, and visit a biological/holistic
>   dentist regularly. Early detection is key.

➢ As with other disease-risk-mitigation efforts, lower
your stress.

CHAPTER 2

YOUR GUT MICROBIOME:
Digest This

THE BODY HAS SEVERAL MICROBIOMES (gut, skin, oral, nasal, respiratory tract, and genital tract), but this chapter will focus primarily on the gut microbiome. Per Merriam-Webster, the microbiome is defined as a community of microorganisms (such as bacteria, fungi, and viruses) that inhabit a particular environment and especially the collection of microorganisms living in or on the human body. The term *microbiota* is used to describe various microorganisms. These microorganisms include bacteria, viruses, fungi, and protozoa. These microorganisms affect metabolic function and our immune system and can protect against pathogens.

The state of your gut health affects your daily quality of health. Some scientists consider the microbiome to be such an essential part of our body that they refer to it as an additional organ. In fact, the gut is the largest endocrine gland in the body. Many believe that the gut microbiome is the epicenter of health. Activity in the gut has a systemic effect.

Hippocrates, considered to be the father of medicine, is known to have said, "All diseases begin in the gut."

Lately, the gut microbiome has been the subject of many studies and research. Combined with technological advancements, this research has revealed the profound impact of our gut microbiome on our overall health.

> Every two to three weeks, you generate an entirely new gut lining.

The entire surface of our intestine (called the epithelium) is lined with a single layer of connected cells which act as a barrier between the outside world and the inside of our bodies. An enterocyte is an epithelial cell that lines the villi of the small intestine and continually regenerates.

HUMAN MICROBIOME PROJECT

The National Institutes of Health started the Human Microbiome Project in 2008.[20] The researchers in this project used advanced genetic techniques to sequence all of the genetic material of the gut microbiome. According to these researchers "...more than 10,000 microbial species occupy the human ecosystem."[21] To give another perspective of the magnitude of what we are composed of, we have approximately thirty trillion cells and thirty-nine trillion microbial cells.

THE GUT AND THE IMMUNE SYSTEM

It is important not to fear germs and other bacteria and microbes in our body.

These microbes are thought to be the main driver of our biology and can either promote healing or promote disease. Our body is quite efficient at controlling germs when our immune system is working well. Germs play a significant role in programming our immune system. Bacteria in the gut regulate the immune system and a recent study in rural China found that certain gut bacterial species may be correlated with chronic inflammation while others may be anti-inflammatory. When our gut bacteria are appropriately balanced, our immune system will function well. When our gut bacteria are unbalanced with an abundance of pathogenic bacteria, the immune system can become overly inflamed and result in gut dysbiosis.[22]

> Research reveals that nearly 90 percent of the cells in our body are bacteria. Many of them are beneficial. Approximately 20 percent of bacterium is pathogenic. The key is to maintain a balance of both good and bad microbes.

Another study published in *Nature*[23] shows how the gut trains the immune system to protect the brain. Dorian McGavern, PhD, one of the authors of the study, states that "this finding opens a new area of neuroimmunology, showing that gut-educated antibody-producing cells inhabit and defend regions that surround the central nervous system."

Exposure to microbes builds strength in one's immune system. Years ago, children played in the dirt often and there was a lower incidence of certain illnesses. There is a concept called the "hygiene hypothesis" which states that lack of early childhood exposure to a diversity of germs can thwart the development of the immune system and result in increased susceptibility to allergies and asthma. Anne Sperling, an immunologist at the University of Chicago, states, "Kids who live in just a bit dirtier environments are actually more protected against asthma and allergies."

DYSBIOSIS

> Dysbiosis refers to an imbalance of good versus bad bacteria and leads to dysfunction in many areas of the body. Abnormal gut flora, or dysbiosis, is a global phenomenon.

When we experience an immune deficiency, dysbiosis results.

Andreas Bäumler, a microbiologist at UC Davis, considers the gut microbiome to be an arm of the immune system whose job is to keep invading pathogens out. He defines dysbiosis functionally as the failure of the immune arm to protect the host, regardless of which bacteria species are present. There are several reasons and as many theories as to how and why the gut becomes dysbiotic. One current theory suggests that modern hygiene practices, including the overuse of antibiotics and improved sanitation, have adversely affected our gut health. Additionally, many other lifestyle choices such as too much alcohol consumption, stress (both emotional and physical), inadequate sleep, a diet lacking in nutrients, and use of too many NSAIDs (non-steroidal anti-inflammatory drugs), and other medications hurt the gut lining and create an imbalance of microbes.

THE ENTERIC NERVOUS SYSTEM: THE REAL BRAIN IS YOUR GUT

Your gut microbiome reflects what you eat, when you eat, and how you eat. There are five stages of human digestion. Before describing the different stages of digestion, it is important to note that all aspects of digestion, including breaking down food, absorbing nutrients, and expelling waste, are regulated by the enteric nervous system. The enteric nervous system is thought of as a digestive brain, and it operates independently of the brain and the spinal cord. The simple act of anticipating eating can release digestive enzymes into the stomach even before you take your first bite of food. Digestion sends signals to the immune system. It is crucial to optimal health to effectively absorb nutrients from the food you consume. Absorption depends on the current health of the gut microbiome. The process of digestion can affect your hormones, skin, sleep, thyroid, metabolism, brain health, and your mood.

THE FIVE STAGES OF DIGESTION

STAGE ONE
The first stage of digestion is Ingestion. This happens when we put food into our mouths. Saliva and the salivary glands under our tongue begin the process of breaking down the food. During this initial stage, we swallow the food, and with waves of involuntary muscular contractions, called peristalsis, the food is pushed through the esophagus.

STAGE TWO
The next phase is Chemical Digestion. As the food moves through the esophagus on its way to the stomach, it mixes with gastric juices. The combination of thorough chewing, saliva, and enzymes all contribute to good digestion. Hydrochloric acid (HCL) and pepsin break down the protein into amino acids. There is a compelling argument for supplementation because cooking removes a lot of enzymes that are necessary for good digestion. Also, as we age, our enzyme production declines and the process of digestion slows down. At this second stage, bacteria and pathogens are killed and the food turns into a substance called *chyme*.

STAGE THREE
The next stage is further Chemical Digestion but at a different level. During this phase, the chyme travels into the upper part of the small intestine, known as the duodenum. It is at this point that

the pancreas releases sodium bicarbonate to neutralize the chyme. An enzyme called amylase is released to break down carbohydrates. The liver secretes a liquid known as bile which is stored in the gall-bladder. The gallbladder releases bile when food reaches the duodenum. Bile is responsible for emulsifying fats and the enzyme called lipase assists in the breakdown of fat. Throughout this phase, muscular contractions facilitate the continued movement into the large intestine.

STAGE FOUR

The fourth stage is Absorption. As the food travels, millions of micro-villi help with the absorption of nutrients into the bloodstream. These microvilli are cellular extensions like microscopic hairs that are responsible for nutrient absorption in the gastrointestinal tract. Studies have concluded that the appropriate balance of good bacteria helps nutrient absorption. There is no shortage of recommendations for taking probiotics to assist in this stage of digestion. I believe that it is ill advised to randomly take probiotics, but I will go into this further in chapter 15. It is quite likely that probiotics may be helpful but should not be taken without identifying your gut microbiome status.

STAGE FIVE

The fifth and final stage of digestion is Elimination. During this phase, undigested food, or food that can't be broken down or absorbed, needs to be eliminated. This food enters the colon and is stored in the rectum which is the last part of the large intestine. The rectum relies on peristalsis (the involuntary constriction and relaxation of the muscles of the intestine) to eliminate this undigested food as the final stage of the digestive process.

This process of digestion is essential to one's overall health. As the gut becomes out of balance, the digestive system becomes a major source of toxicity and releases toxins into the bloodstream.

IT'S NOT ONLY WHAT YOU EAT, IT'S WHEN YOU EAT

When you eat has recently become an interesting topic. Among other authors, Satchin Panda has written a book, called *The Circadian Code*, all about the circadian clocks which are the programs that control our daily rhythms. I will cover this fascinating information in depth in chapter 14, but it bears noting that the timing of our eating has a great impact on our overall health. I will also repeat throughout this book that circadian biology is a material concept to grasp when optimizing one's health. Scientists have discovered that a group of immune cells important for regulating the health of the gut microbiome is tied to circadian rhythms. When the timing of your food consumption is inconsistent or during late hours, your gut can suffer. These cells are called group 3 innate lymphoid cells, and they help maintain a healthy balance among bacteria and the gut. There are several studies showing fasting can fix your metabolism and that time-restricted eating (within eight to twelve hours) reduces the incidence of chronic disease. These studies further conclude that 90 percent of all chronic disease has been connected to the microbiome. Diet both feeds and influences the microbes in our gut.

THE HADZA IN TANZANIA HAVE IT RIGHT

The food you choose to eat affects the diversity of your gut microbiome which will, in turn, affect your immune system, central nervous system, brain function, and likely your heart health.

There have been many studies on the Hadza people in Tanzania to learn about the importance of gut microbial diversity. These people only eat what they find in the wild and they are extraordinarily "gut healthy." The Hadza people have about 40 percent higher gut diversity than most Americans. They consume nearly six hundred species of plants and animals in a year as opposed to the fifty species that Americans consume. It is noteworthy that the Hadza people have little or no obesity, allergies, cardiovascular disease, or cancer while these diseases plague Western culture. It is thought that our Western diet is responsible for the decline in microbial diversity and that diversity is essential to our well-being.

One striking difference was the amount of fiber that the Hadza eat in comparison to the consumption of fiber by those of us in the West. According to Justin Sonnenburg, PhD, a professor at Stanford University, "the Hadza get 100 or more grams of fiber a day in their food, on average. We [in the West] average 15 grams per day."[24]

There are two kinds of fiber. Recommendations indicate that one needs to consume between twenty-five to forty grams per day as opposed to the ten to fifteen grams that most of us get. Soluble fiber dissolves in water, slows the digestive process, and lowers cholesterol. It is also thought to stabilize blood sugar and feed healthy gut bacteria. Soluble fiber expands in your stomach and can give you a feeling of satiety. Examples of soluble-fiber foods are beans, seeds, peas, barley, oat bran, and some fruits and vegetables. Insoluble fiber does not dissolve in water and remains intact as it travels through the gastrointestinal tract. Its benefits include preventing constipation, slowing down the absorption of carbohydrates, and preventing certain gastrointestinal issues. Examples of foods containing insoluble fiber include seeds, fruit peels, whole wheat bread, avocado, spinach, potatoes, almonds, walnuts, and brown rice.

A diverse diet is important to maintain the necessary gut microbial diversity.

Routinized eating, which I have been an offender of, is easy and time efficient but not ideal for optimal health. For years, before I knew better, I ate the same thing for breakfast and for lunch. I did vary my dinner choices, but only among three different foods. I know now that I was not doing my gut microbiome any favors. Currently, there are some recommendations that eating twenty-five to thirty different species of plants will aid in increasing your microbial diversity. There was a study published that concluded that everyone's collection of microbes varies in both number as well as diversity of species. It also stated that the healthiest among us has the most plentiful and diverse bacteria.[25] A healthy microbiome impacts our general health, gut health, and mental health. The higher the microbial diversity people have, the healthier they are. Many chronic diseases are associated with low microbial diversity.

The food you eat controls your blood sugar and can either lower or raise your risk of diabetes. High fiber, in general, tends to be better for your gut and increases microbial diversity. Examples of food choices impacting your gut include the inflammation that can result from consumption of both wheat and dairy, the havoc that artificial sweeteners can wreak on your gut, the increase in microbes that love to feed on sugar which results in *Candida* due to a diet high in sugar, and the alteration of one's microbiome caused by eating GMO foods that have been sprayed with glyphosate to make them resistant to pests. There are many who would object to the elimination of dairy and wheat from your diet. The best approach is to determine what works best for you and your own biochemistry and genetics. If wheat and dairy work well for you and do not cause you any obvious discomfort, then continue consuming both. I would suggest that you do at least one test to reveal your internal state and any subtle reactions you may have to particular foods. The test which I like the best is called the GI Effects Comprehensive Stool Profile by Genova Diagnostics. I also suggest that if you choose to consume wheat and dairy, you should make every effort to get organic, hormone- and antibiotic-free products. Nutritional science is among the areas of science with the most conflict. One can find as many studies as to why eggs, coffee, wine, and so on are great for you as there are studies concluding the harmful effects of consuming these different things. Another reason for the great deal of conflict in nutritional science is that different people metabolize the same foods in highly individualized ways. Despite the ongoing controversy regarding what foods are best to eat, it is uncontroverted that the worst foods you can eat are processed foods ladened with sugar.

MY STORY

About five years ago when I felt it was time to pay close attention to my health and my habits, I found a functional medicine doctor located in Northern California. He had a long waiting list to see him, but when I finally got in, I had to take about eight different tests prior to my first appointment. It required three months, a spreadsheet, and a precision strategy to figure out what I could eat, what I had to eat, and what I couldn't eat in order to get accurate results from all of the tests. When I traveled to see him from my home in Southern California, I was curious to learn about the results of my tests. The first thing he said to me was that I had serious celiac disease and three different tests confirmed this condition. I was beyond surprised to hear this since gluten had been one of my favorite food groups (along with sugar) for most of my life. I freely admit that I had the eating habits of a twelve-year-old. I did not like any green food tainting my plate. The reality was that I had no idea of the damage that I was experiencing internally. I even questioned how I could have celiac disease since I never experienced stomachaches or any kind of discomfort from my poor diet. The doctor explained that celiac disease, gluten intolerance, and gluten sensitivity, all variations of the same issue, manifested in a variety of ways. Some people with this issue experienced stomachaches, some had skin rashes, and others had brain inflammation. I had neither stomachaches nor skin rashes, but I realized that brain inflammation is a subtle problem that has symptoms that can be confused with aging, lack of sleep, and other more benign explanations. I was particularly horrified since my father was in the throes of devastating cognitive decline. I wondered if his diet could have been a contributing factor to his disease and ultimate death. The doctor said to me, "If I were you, I would never eat anything containing gluten for the rest of my life." Motivated by a strong desire to avoid brain inflammation or any neurodegenerative disease, I have avoided gluten since the day I walked out of that doctor's office. I feel more energetic and have less brain fog. I don't know if that is attributable to my gluten avoidance or due to one or a combination of the many other lifestyle alterations I have done. In any event, I am delighted to feel better.

GUT AND CHRONIC DISEASE

One way that the microbiome contributes to Alzheimer's disease, cardiovascular disease, and many other chronic diseases is the presence of lipopolysaccharides. Known as LPS for short, these are molecules that are endotoxins. Endotoxins are a type of bacterial toxin that is in the cell wall of gram-negative bacteria. The definition of *endotoxin* is "a poison that is produced by and remains inside a living cell."[26] These toxins can be diet induced, and once released, destroy tissues, trigger an immune response, and cause inflammation.[27],[28] Endotoxins, along with protein fragments, bacteria, and waste, pass through the gut lining when the tight junctions binding the enterocyte cells become "leaky." This is referred to as intestinal permeability, or leaky gut, and contributes to a decline in absorption and increased inflammation. When your gut becomes leaky or your intestinal wall becomes permeable, this is called "barrier disintegrity" and is something to be avoided. When barrier disintegrity begins, deleterious compounds can enter one's systemic circulation.

Another kind of "poison" is artificial sweeteners. These are known to disrupt the metabolism of microbes and reduce gut diversity. Artificial sweeteners cause glucose intolerance by adversely altering the gut microbiome. Using these artificial sweeteners has been associated with obesity, metabolic dysfunction, and other chronic diseases.[29]

Antibiotics are responsible for saving many lives and have been nothing short of miraculous in many instances. However, they are also egregiously overprescribed. The overprescribing of antibiotics has not only led to serious antibiotic-resistant infections but also has had a deleterious impact on our gut microbiome. When we consume antibiotics, they act like indeterminate destroyers. They destroy both bad and good bacteria. While I am not suggesting that you should avoid taking antibiotics when there is a real need for them, you should be judicious in your consumption.

It is thought that Alzheimer's disease may start in the gut and spread to the brain. People who have died from Alzheimer's disease have been found to have beta-amyloid deposits in their gut. This beta-amyloid is a protein that forms plaque in the brain which is thought to be a contributing cause of neurodegeneration.

There is a direct connection between the gut and the brain. Through one's neuronal pathways and through cytokines (chemical messengers), our brain chemistry is affected by our gut. While the mechanism of this action is complicated, the simple explanation is that the gut and the brain communicate with each other. There are countless studies about the connections between the bacteria in your gut and one's mood and anxiety levels. There are also direct connections between one's gut and their liver, their lungs, and their kidneys. It appears to be imperative to maintain optimal gut health to avoid chronic disease and maintain good health.

THE VAGUS NERVE CONNECTS YOUR TWO BRAINS

Stress, anxiety, depression, and negative emotions can decrease your brain activity which in turn decreases activation of the vagus nerve. The vagus nerve is the longest nerve of the autonomic nervous system in the human body and runs from the brain stem all the way down through the neck and into the chest and abdomen. There are more neurotransmitters in the gut than there are in the brain.

It is thought that stress can make the gut more vulnerable to infection. The innate immune system is located primarily in the gut, and it is the first line of defense.[30] Stress can cause a cascade of responses that slows down your digestive functions. Pancreatic enzymes decline in production, gallbladder function declines, stomach acid production declines, gut motility decreases, and ultimately the intestinal immune system is suppressed.

The brain and the gut have a bidirectional relationship. They are in constant communication via the vagus nerve. This nerve is responsible for the function of the heart, lungs, and digestive tract. Our state of mind affects the state of our gut and vice versa.

EXERCISE AND THE GUT

It is thought that the effect of exercise on the gut microbiome is beneficial to overall health. Consistent exercise increases the gut microbes which assist in the production of short-chain fatty acids. This is important because short-chain fatty acids lower one's risk of inflammatory diseases.[31] There has been an abundance of research conducted on the impact of exercise on gut barrier integrity, immune regulation, and reduction in inflammation. Gut improvement is just one more reason to establish a consistent exercise routine. There are many other reasons which will be discussed in chapter 8 on movement.

BRAIN-SKIN-GUT CONNECTION

Another interesting bidirectional relationship is that of gastrointestinal health and skin status. The connection has not yet been defined with complete certainty and there are several theories attempting to make sense of this axis. The brain-gut-skin connection was originally conceived by John H. Stokes and Donald M. Pillsbury in 1930. They hypothesized that "negative emotional states such as depression and anxiety alter the gastrointestinal function and lead to changes in normal gut flora, increased intestinal permeability, and systemic inflammation."[32] While science has advanced in many sophisticated ways since the 1930s, many aspects of the Stokes-Pillsbury theory have been validated.[33] The most likely explanation for this relationship is neurologic and immunologic responses which result in chronic systemic inflammation.

EXERCISE CAUTION IN SELF-TREATING

There are several nutrients and supplements that can help treat the leaky gut problem caused by endotoxins and other pathogens entering the bloodstream. Zinc, quercetin, butyrate, curcumin, indole, berberine, and DGL (deglycyrrhizinated licorice) have all been shown to regulate permeability and strengthen the gut barrier. Each one of these modulates the issue in different ways, and it's best to determine your own particular issue before taking anything. You should also exercise caution when taking the ubiquitously prescribed probiotics.

They are widely recommended but should not be taken randomly without first identifying through testing the source of your dysbiosis, or unbalanced gut bacteria. Each different probiotic contains millions of different strains and species of bacteria. Different strains and species have different effects. If you have dysbiosis (which most of us do to some degree), you have an overabundance of certain bacteria and microbes, and it is unwise to inadvertently take the wrong probiotic, which could add to the imbalance. You need to identify which bacteria you are deficient in or overloaded with and choose your probiotic accordingly.

While there is still a great deal that is unknown about the microbiome, a further understanding of the connection between the microbiome and disease will be valuable in identifying both treatment and preventive protocols to improve health. It is becoming clear that the gut microbiome is influenced by many different factors. Several microbe-related therapeutics focused on neurodegeneration, cancer, and other diseases will hit the market soon.

ACTION STEPS

- ➤ Increase the diversity in your diet.
- ➤ Increase your fiber intake.
- ➤ Avoid snacking between meals.
- ➤ Avoid artificial sweeteners.
- ➤ Only take antibiotics when there is no alternative method of healing.
- ➤ Eat a lot of vegetables, fruits, legumes, and beans.
- ➤ Eat fermented foods.

CHAPTER 3

IMMUNITY and INFLAMMATION:
Get to Know Your Most Powerful Ally

SIMPLY PUT, OUR IMMUNE SYSTEM protects us from harmful invaders and the process of inflammation communicates to our organs the messages of the immune system. This system enables us to respond to the many threats from our environment. As we age, our immune system loses function and renders us vulnerable to infections, cancer, and autoimmune disease. Exposure to toxins and viruses also contributes to the overall immune system decline.

> An optimal immune system is the key to good health and longevity.

IMMUNE CELLS

The cells of the immune system are found throughout the body in the bone marrow, skin, thymus gland, spleen, lymph nodes, tonsils, liver, and gut. Immune cells are also known as white blood cells or leukocytes. There are eight types of white blood cells: macrophages, dendritic cells, neutrophils, eosinophils, basophils, T cells, B cells, and natural killer cells (NK cells).

TWO-PART IMMUNE SYSTEM

IMMUNE SENESCENCE

As we age, our natural killer cells, whose function is to fight against infections and cancer, become inefficient at their job which gives way to "immune senescence." This immune senescence is considered the leading cause of disability and death as we get older.

Natural killer cells are our body's first defense against viruses and cancer cells, and they are a fundamental part of the first of the body's two-part immune system, the "innate immune system." The job of these killer cells is to slow the growth or kill off infected cells or tumor cells. In the event the innate immune system is unable to extinguish the threat, the second part of the immune system, the "adaptive immune system," takes over. This second phase is a result of a lifetime of exposure to different pathogens and produces antibodies called B cells to respond to the threat. The defining feature of the adaptive immune system is its memory. It remembers pathogens and increases resilience to subsequent threats. The reaction to a pathogen informs how sick you become. If the pathogen is familiar to your system, you will likely get rid of it in a few days and feel better. If the threat is from an unknown or unfamiliar pathogen, it can take weeks to mount an effective defense. Usually, a healthy immune response will defeat the threat and shut itself off. Sometimes, one's body overreacts and cannot shut off the immune response when necessary and triggers a "cytokine storm." This is an indication of a dangerous systemic inflammatory response. It is not precisely known why this happens to some people and not to others, although genetic factors are likely involved.

INTEGUMENTARY SYSTEM

Your integumentary system is defined as skin, hair, nails, glands, and nerves. This system acts to protect you from external threats including bacteria, viruses, pathogens, infection, chemical assault, and radiation damage. To optimize this important line of defense, you need to clean this microbiome with regular soap and water. Under most circumstances, constant use of antibacterial soap is ill advised. We now know the perils of overusing antibiotics include eliminating all of the good bacteria along with the bad. Frequent use of antibacterial soaps and wipes does the same thing. It kills both the good and the bad bacteria indiscriminately.

When you encounter harmful bacteria, your immune system kicks into action. The first step is the release of chemicals that hold off the pathogens. The next step is the release of macrophages, which are cells that destroy the bacteria and communicate to the rest of the immune system that it is time to shift into response gear. When this communication occurs, increased blood flow is sent to the area of infection. White blood cells attack the offending bacteria and cause cell division to heal damaged tissues. This last step triggers inflammation.

While it is generally thought that getting sick can strengthen your immune system, hence the phrase "that which does not kill me makes me stronger," recent research reveals that contracting the measles virus wipes out the immune system's memory and over 70 percent of its antibodies. So, instead of becoming stronger after enduring measles, you become more vulnerable to other infections. The same research has shown that a measles vaccine that prevents contracting the disease provides important protection of the immune system by preventing this memory loss.[34],[35] There is also interesting research, though not definitive, that influenza and other viral infections can contribute to neurodegeneration. It is possible, and may be explained by an individual response, that the pro-inflammatory antibody proteins called cytokines which are released to fight the pathogens may impact the central nervous system and the brain and disrupt the normal functioning of neurotransmitters.

AUTOIMMUNITY

I suffer from environmental allergies and often wonder why my immune system misinterprets seemingly nonthreatening things like grass, pollen, and trees as a threat to my well-being and causes a very annoying reaction of itchy eyes, sneezing, and a perpetually runny nose. Far more severe autoimmune diseases like lupus, multiple sclerosis, and rheumatoid arthritis result in the immune system attacking one's cells and tissues. These widespread disorders are not completely understood but are thought to be caused by genetics, environment, infections, and even medication reactions.

One's immune system dysfunction can either be underactive or overactive. When an immune system is overactive, autoimmune disease results. Autoimmunity is when your body mounts a misdirected immune response to an otherwise benign invader. An example of this is allergies.

GERM THEORY

When researching immunity, I came across the conflicting theories of germ theory and terrain theory. Germ theory was proposed by Louis Pasteur, who lived in the 1800s. He was known as one of the fathers of germ theory even though variations of this theory have existed since ancient times. Germ theory is what has been most widely accepted by mainstream medicine and states that germs, including bacteria, fungi, and viruses, invade the body and cause disease. The focus is on killing the germs by nearly any means necessary. Methods include antibiotics, chemotherapy, surgery, and anything focused on eradicating something external which has invaded the body.

TERRAIN THEORY

Antoine Béchamp was another French scientific researcher who studied disease pathology and lived in the nineteenth century. He proposed a theory known as the "terrain theory," or the cellular theory, and it stated that our internal health is responsible for whether we get sick. He said that the state of the microorganisms inside our cells and tissues will determine our health and that disease is a result of a weakened immune system. He said that "the primary cause of disease is in us, always in us." While germ theory emphasizes drugs and external solutions, terrain theory emphasizes cell health and immune system strength. Terrain theory has largely been ignored by conventional medicine but has been embraced by functional medicine, traditional Chinese medicine, and other natural healing methods. These branches of medicine highlight detoxification, nutrition, and other lifestyle choices to create internal health.

IS THE OVERZEALOUS KILLING OF GERMS THE RIGHT APPROACH?

A clear drawback of prioritizing killing germs is the overuse of antibiotics and the resulting rise of superbugs and infections that are antibiotic resistant. Another drawback of the overemphasis of sterilization, disinfecting everything, and heavy antibiotic use is that it has made us more susceptible to infection and illness. There are many anecdotal stories of children playing in the dirt generations ago and ending up being healthier and more resilient than kids today who are always doused with antibacterial soap and have a higher incidence of asthma and allergies. During the COVID-19 pandemic, the vast range of individual responses to the virus was explained by the underlying health of the patient. There are of course exceptions, and we still don't understand why some seemingly healthy people had drastic reactions, but, by and large, patients with preexisting conditions had far more serious reactions. Like everything else, behavior somewhere in the middle of the two theories probably represents the most sensible approach.

THE KEY IS TO MODULATE YOUR IMMUNE SYSTEM

There are several ways to modulate your immune system and reduce your susceptibility to disease. It is critical to understand the concept of autophagy.

As we age and our cells go through continuous division, they become damaged, or what is called "senescent." A senescent cell has lost the ability to reproduce, stops dividing, but remains metabolically active. Ideally, we need these cells to be removed from our body so they can't do damage or contribute to disease. An interesting element of this is another concept called the "Hayflick Limit." Leonard Hayflick, PhD, a professor of anatomy at the UCSF School of Medicine, discovered that cells have a maximum number of fifty divisions before becoming senescent. Autophagic dysfunction is associated with many diseases and, in 2016, Yoshinori Ohsumi won the Nobel Prize in Physiology or Medicine for his discoveries of the mechanisms for autophagy. He noted that some of the functions of autophagy include the prevention of genotoxic stress, tumor suppression, pathogen elimination,

> The word autophagy is derived from ancient Greek language that means "self-devouring" or "eating of self."[197] It describes the process in which cellular waste and dysfunctional proteins are cleared away and recycled and it is essential to good health.

regulation of immunity and inflammation, metabolism, and cellular survival. An imbalanced autophagy is a driver of premature aging and restoring balanced autophagy is essential to slowing the aging process. This process declines as we age, like so many others, and when the dysfunctional cells and toxic proteins aren't removed, they can multiply, do harm, and trigger disease. You can facilitate autophagy by intermittent fasting, exercise, and cold and heat exposure. When you fast, you free up enzyme potential to focus on healing instead of on digesting. Even time-restricted eating reduces inflammation and improves immune function. Exercise stimulates lymph fluid and immunity. Heat exposure allows for the elimination of heavy metals and toxins. Cold exposure increases the production of glutathione which is the body's main antioxidant and is produced in the liver. Glutathione enhances the activity of the immune cells and provides protection from free radicals. In addition, quality of sleep and stress reduction all increase resilience and modulate the immune system. Both sleep and the immune system are regulated by circadian clocks. It is becoming widely accepted that balancing your autonomic nervous system can help optimize your health. Improving your gut microbiome will go a long way to benefitting your immune system, as so many immune cells reside in the gut.

STRESS AND YOUR IMMUNE SYSTEM

During periods of stress, your immune system responds by triggering an inflammatory response. If this inflammatory response is acute, or short lived, it can be helpful. If the inflammation continues and becomes chronic, a path to chronic disease begins.

Your immune system is aware when you are under stress. "While long-term stress is generally harmful, short-term stress can be protective as it prepares the organism to deal with challenges."[36]

Studies have been performed on medical students during their exams. The results were declining numbers of natural killer cells and T cells. Other studies found that older people who were already in declining health were more susceptible to stress-related immunity decline.[37]

FOOD AND YOUR IMMUNE SYSTEM

A nutrient-dense diet is an important step to enhancing immunity. *Eat to Beat Disease* by Dr. William Li lists specific foods which can boost immune function. I will reference the foods that he highlights but suggest you read this book for a more comprehensive explanation.

There are foods that boost immune function and foods which can turn down or calm an overactive immune response. First, I will cover the immune-boosting foods. While there is research suggesting the enormous benefits of most mushrooms, the white button mushroom has been studied the most for its immune-stimulating benefits.

The members of the allium family, onions, leeks, and shallots, all have been shown to increase glutathione levels and immune response. Garlic and, in particular, aged garlic contains an ingredient called apigenin which increases immune T cells and natural killer cells.

Broccoli sprouts contain an ingredient called sulforaphane which is found at a far greater concentration in broccoli sprouts than in regular broccoli. It increases natural killer cells.

Extra-virgin olive oil contains hydroxytyrosol, oleocanthal, and oleic acid. While the source of the olive oil is critical because the benefits vary according to where it comes from and how it was made, if high quality, it boosts immune function and decreases inflammation. Studies have shown that it increases immune T cells and even reduces the body's reaction to allergies.

A substance called ellagic acid, found in walnuts, chestnuts, blackberries, black raspberries, and pomegranates, improves the ability of immune cells to detect and destroy cancer cells.

You need to be wary of the high sugar content in fruit juices because spikes in blood sugar adversely impact your immune system. If consumed occasionally, cranberry juice increases T cells and is known to activate the immune system throughout your body, not just your bladder. Concord grape juice contains anthocyanins, procyanidins, and hydroxycinnamic acid, which provide DNA protection and immune-boosting benefits.

Blueberries increase myeloid dendritic cells and natural killer cells and decrease inflammation while increasing immune function. Elderberries and other dark berries have polyphenols and antioxidants that modulate the gut microbiome and improve immunity.

Chili peppers contain capsaicin, which activates the immune system and increases white blood cells and B cells.

Pacific oysters contain immune-stimulating peptides and are DNA protective. They increase natural killer cells and are anti-inflammatory.

Licorice (the root, not the candy) contains glycyrrhetinic acid which improves immune response. It should only be used in moderation because of its potential to alter sodium and potassium levels.

Eggs, beef, dark leafy greens, and cruciferous vegetables increase the production of glutathione, which is essential for optimal immunity. Many in the world of nutrition espouse the theory that one should "eat head to tail" for maximum nutrient density. This includes eating liver, kidney, and heart. I cannot weigh in on this because I am just not capable of eating that way.

Raw honey and bee pollen both strengthen the immune system and inhibit pathogen growth. They are inherently antimicrobial but cannot be given to infants.

There are many herbs and spices which have been found to have powerful immune benefits. These include dandelion, chamomile, ginseng, echinacea, winter cherry, ginkgo biloba, astragalus, cat's-claw, garlic, ginger, turmeric, thyme, rosemary, clove, and lemon balm.

Many foods that contain vitamin C may calm down an overactive immune system and can be a part of an autoimmune protocol. Vitamin C has been found to be beneficial for an overactive immune system. Some of these foods include acerola, broccoli, camu camu, cherry tomato, guava, oranges, and strawberries. Also, green tea which contains EGCG (epigallocatechin-3-gallate) lowers the number of pro-inflammatory T cells and can modulate the immune system to quell overactivity.

TAKING SUPPLEMENTS

If they discuss nutrition with you at all, most conventional doctors will tell you to get your nutrients only from food. That would be ideal in a perfect world, but we don't live in that world. We live in a world, particularly in the US, where the soil has been depleted of minerals, the food supply has been tainted with pesticides, and as we age we lose important enzymes for efficient digestion. Therefore, taking supplements, while controversial, is a necessary part of one's quest for optimal health.

VITAMIN C

The research about the health benefits of vitamin C is conflicting. In 1954, Linus Pauling won the Nobel Prize in Chemistry. He conducted many studies on vitamin C and its ability to boost the immune system. Subsequent studies refuted claims that large doses of vitamin C could prevent the common cold and concluded that the vitamin could only shorten the duration of the cold. There are also studies that specifically confirm that "vitamin C contributes to immune defense by supporting various cellular functions of both the innate and the adaptive immune system."[38] Dr. Li explains that vitamin C affects the immune system by increasing the body's production of regulatory T cells, or Treg cells. These cells modulate the immune system and aid in achieving a balance between an underactive and an overactive system.

VITAMIN D

Vitamin D plays an important role in both the innate and adaptive immune systems. Studies have concluded that deficiencies in vitamin D are associated with increased autoimmunity and susceptibility to infection.[39] Not only are there many books, articles, and studies on vitamin D, during the COVID pandemic, monitoring one's levels of this vitamin (which is in fact a hormone) is one of the few agreed-upon protocols. My research has revealed that you should not just randomly take vitamin D on your own without first finding out about your serum levels. It is also advised to monitor levels of other vitamins, like A, because these impact one another. Whenever you're taking vitamin D3, it is essential to take it with vitamin K2 to prevent improper circulating and calcification.

SELENIUM

Selenium is a micronutrient that is required for immune system health. It increases cellular immune response and helps with the production of T cells.[40]

ZINC

Zinc is a mineral that is involved in many biological processes, but its most important role pertains to the immune system. It aids in both the growth and the function of immune cells. If you have sufficient zinc levels in your body, your immune system will function better, but if you are deficient in this mineral, you will be more susceptible to disease. It is advised to seek advice as to appropriate doses because excessive doses can alter your copper levels.

MUSHROOMS

Reishi mushrooms are referred to as "medicinal mushrooms" and have been studied for their health benefits. A 2006 study showed that reishi mushrooms are immune system modulators and can both stimulate and calm the immune system when necessary. They have been found to grow and strengthen T and B cells.[41]

MELATONIN

Melatonin is a hormone, and we have melatonin receptors through-out our body. As our endogenous production of melatonin declines with age, there is a direct association with the age-related decline of the functioning of our immune system. Melatonin acts as an immune system modulator in that it stimulates immunity when needed and suppresses immunity when needed. Its benefit is connected to its influence on circadian rhythms which impact the immune system.[42] I think it's prudent to begin with a very low dose (0.5 mg) and increase according to your response.

Two additional modes of supporting immunity include the use of Cistanche and lactoferrin. Cistanche is a desert plant that has been used in Eastern medicine for a long time. It is thought to have great antioxidant properties and to support immunity. Lactoferrin is a protein found in both cow's milk and human milk. It is antiox-idant, antibacterial, antifungal, antiparasitic, and antiviral, and its function is to transport and bind iron ions within the immune sys-tem. It is a newborn's first defense against the world and is known to be beneficial beyond infancy.[43]

PHOTOBIOMODULATION AND YOUR IMMUNE SYSTEM

Light technology involving red light, blue light, and ultraviolet light have all been shown to have significant therapeutic potential in terms of optimizing one's immune system.[44] Light therapy is discussed in detail in the chapter on light optimization. I don't know why mainstream medicine has not embraced this form of therapy, as it has been shown to improve the health and resilience of cells and tissues and is extremely safe. It has been safe for years in treating illness. In 1903, Dr. Niels Ryberg Finsen received the Nobel Prize in Physiology or Medicine for successfully treating tuberculosis with ultraviolet or blue light and for treating smallpox with red light and, since then, many studies have shown that this therapy can improve immune function and reduce inflammation. The mechanism of action is thought to be from increasing nitric oxide and increasing ATP and optimizing mitochondria.[45] "Many studies have demonstrated that PBM [photobiomodulation] modulates inflammation by reducing pro-inflammatory cytokines [...] and other inflammatory markers released from activated inflammatory cells, while increasing the anti-inflammatory cytokines [...]."[46]

COLD THERAPY

In chapter 11, I will explain in detail the benefits of this type of therapy. Brief exposure to cold can stimulate your immune system. Like light therapy, cold therapy has also been used therapeutically for ages. Hippocrates, the father of medicine, is said to have used cold water in his treatment of illness. Short periods of cold exposure increase T lymphocytes and natural killer cells. It also increases metabolic rate and stimulates vasodilation and vasoconstriction which improves your circulation and lymph flow. Finally, this process increases white blood cell count and decreases inflammation. After a brief cold shower, the body begins the process of warming itself. As the warming begins, your metabolic rate increases, the immune system is triggered, and more white blood cells are released which protect you from illness. However, if you have heart issues, proceed with caution as the studies show that cold therapy has the potential to cause transient arrhythmias.[47]

THE CONNECTION BETWEEN THE IMMUNE SYSTEM AND INFLAMMATION

The immune system and inflammation are intricately connected. The immune system needs an appropriate number of stressors to maintain homeostasis. Inflammation is an immune response that stimulates cell regeneration. The key is balance. While we are bombarded with information about reducing inflammation as the key to avoiding disease, you can't decrease inflammation without suppressing the immune system in some way. If you embark on a path that includes too many anti-inflammatory therapies, you will increase the likelihood of illness.

ACUTE VS. CHRONIC INFLAMMATION

The combined effect of the accumulation of old cells and the inability to produce new cells increases inflammation. There is a concept just recently given the name "inflammazone." This term was developed in 2002 by Dr. Jürg Tschopp to describe a group of molecules that are responsible for the governing of the inflammatory response.

TEST YOUR INFLAMMATORY BIOMARKERS

Obesity, Alzheimer's disease, type 2 diabetes, cancer, and cardiovascular disease are all driven by chronic inflammation. An insidious aspect of chronic inflammation is that it is silent and one often is

There is an important distinction between acute and chronic inflammation. We must have the process of acute inflammation as it promotes healing when our body is faced with a threat. Without our immune system triggering acute inflammation, we would not heal. It is lifesaving. The problem arises when the immune system fails to shut off as it is designed to do after the initial response. When the inflammation continues, it becomes chronic and is the foundation of every chronic disease.

unaware of its presence. There are many testing options available to measure your level of inflammation, and it's prudent to track these biomarkers. Some of the most important inflammatory lab markers include hs-CRP, HbA1C, fasting insulin, serum ferritin, red blood cell distribution width, homocysteine, ESR and platelets, lactate dehydrogenase (LDH), neutrophil to lymphocyte ratio (NLR), liver enzymes, lipid panel, and vitamin D3. Symptoms of chronic inflammation include aches and pains, skin issues, digestive discomfort, memory impairment, elevated CRP, and cholesterol imbalance. As inflammation persists, cells, organs, and blood vessels become damaged and lose function.

INFLAMMAGING

While many of the causes of chronic inflammation include poor diet, poor sleep quality, smoking, environmental toxins, stress, and even genetics, age is a factor that has recently garnered a great deal of attention. As we age, our immune cells become less responsive and ultimately ineffective.

Scientists have coined a term called "inflammaging" to describe the process of age-related inflammation. It is a low-grade, unresolved inflammation.

As we age, the function of our T cells declines and their ability to fight pathogens weakens. The result of this is that many elderly people become more susceptible to infections and less responsive to vaccinations. The T cells lose function because our mitochondria begin to malfunction. As these T cells decline, they release inflammatory-stimulating molecules, promoting chronic inflammation, damaging tissues, and leading to age-related diseases.[48]

Exercise has a paradoxical effect on inflammation. Moderate, consistent exercise reduces inflammation but excessive, endurance exercise is pro-inflammatory. In fact, all exercise is pro-inflammatory while you are in its midst, but if it's a moderate amount, the inflammatory-reducing benefits persist after you are finished exercising.

Smart Choices: Pro and Anti-inflammatory Foods

The Inflammation Research Foundation, founded in 2003 by Dr. Barry Sears, is focused on the relationship between diet and inflammation. Pro-inflammatory foods include all refined carbohydrates (particularly those containing white flour), gluten, sugar and high fructose corn syrup, conventionally raised meat and dairy, farm-raised fish and seafood, processed conventional meats, trans fats (partially hydrogenated oil), food additives and preservatives, highly processed vegetable and seed oils, and artificial sweeteners. Anti-inflammatory foods include berries, wild fatty fish, broccoli, avocados, green tea, peppers (chili and bell), mushrooms, grapes, turmeric, extra-virgin olive oil, dark chocolate, cherries, carrots, tomatoes, almonds, walnuts, oranges, sweet potatoes, and leafy greens like kale, spinach, and Swiss chard. An emerging view is that industrialized vegetable and seed oils like canola, corn, sunflower, cottonseed, and soy are causing the most harm in our diet. They contain high amounts of polyunsaturated fat (PUFAs) which makes them chemically unstable and susceptible to oxidation. Oxidized fats are harmful because they are inflammatory. These oils have a harmful ratio of omega-6s, which are inflammatory, to omega-3s, which are anti-inflammatory.

THE CELL DANGER RESPONSE

When dealing with immunity and inflammation, it's helpful to consider the work of Dr. Robert Naviaux.

Naviaux wrote a paper titled "Metabolic features of the cell danger response,"[198] where he explains the shift in mitochondrial energy that precludes inflammation and disease. When our mitochondria are in a healthy state, they are resilient and able to deal with the threats that come their way. When too many toxins, too much stress, too much exercise, or too poor of a diet bombard our system, a metabolic response is triggered which pushes the body out of homeostasis, impairs organ functioning, stimulates the release of inflammatory cytokines, and paves the way for chronic disease.

This cell danger response is tantamount to being stuck in a fight-or-flight state marked by chronic inflammation. Naviaux believes that this underlies most chronic fatigue symptoms. Ideally, it's best to first identify the trigger of this cell danger response to effectively heal it. When the source is difficult to determine, the protocol is to improve your circadian rhythms and sleep, lower your stress, improve your diet, and eliminate or at least reduce your toxin exposure. I realize how repetitive this must sound, but the reality is that the same four or five lifestyle changes are responsible for optimizing nearly every aspect of your health.

SUPPLEMENTS AND IMMUNITY

There are many anti-inflammatory supplements that are recommended to reduce inflammation. I will briefly list the most frequently suggested ones with the proviso that it is far more nuanced, and you need to be cautious. There is a synergistic effect as well as your very own individual response to consider. N-acetyl cysteine gets a lot of press coverage, along with alpha-lipoic acid. Both are thought to reduce oxidative stress and inflammation. Curcumin is probably the most studied herb/supplement and has a great deal of science supporting its benefits. Resveratrol, ginger, and reishi mushrooms appear to be effective as well. Fish oil or omega-3 fatty acid supplementation has been in favor for a while, but there is some conflicting science about the potential rancidity of the supplements, so proceed with caution.

METFORMIN

Another interesting and emerging drug for reducing inflammation is called metformin. This drug has been around for a long time for the treatment of diabetes, but in the era of "repurposing" drugs, it has been studied for its anti-inflammatory, oxidative stress reduction, and antiaging benefits. Many biohackers and tech entrepreneurs take this drug whether or not they have diabetes in pursuit of antiaging benefits. Despite the existing studies of metformin, more research needs to be conducted to determine the safety and efficacy of this drug. The underlying mechanisms are not well understood, and people tend to have a varied response to taking this drug. If you have liver or kidney issues, you would be wise to steer clear of this method of reducing inflammation. One should exercise caution and prudently source this drug. Recently, there have been numerous recalls of tainted metformin.

Taking steps toward optimizing one's immune system is the best defense we have against this and any future viruses and pandemics. The speed at which the COVID-19 vaccine was developed and distributed was quite remarkable. It may be more complicated or take longer during the next pandemic, so we would be better served to focus on becoming more resilient. It is far more sensible to improve your resilience by optimizing your immune system so you will be able to mount an effective attack against any threat that comes your way.

A suboptimal immune system results in a loss of resilience and an increase in vulnerability to disease. Never forget that your body is constantly responding to everything that you put in it and to everything that you expose it to. Signs of inflammation are quiet and subtle at first. If not mitigated, these signs turn into full-blown disease. While the pursuit of perfect health is an unrealistic goal, focusing on fighting chronic inflammation is a critical step to slowing down the aging process and avoiding disease. While most of us, if we are fortunate to live long enough, will be unable to avoid certain age-related diseases, a reasonable goal is to delay the onset of these diseases for as long as possible. Choosing healthy lifestyle habits will reduce one's susceptibility to inflammation and disease and could reduce the negative effects of aging. An optimal immune system should be a top priority.

ACTION STEPS

➢ Avoid sugar and other pro-inflammatory foods. Various foods trigger inflammation in different people. Determine your triggers.

➢ Test. Get a blood count, metabolic panel, and other inflammatory markers.

➢ Manage your stress. Activate your parasympathetic nervous system, which will optimize your immune system.

➢ Get out in nature for a great immunity boost.

➢ Make sure that your gut is in peak condition.

➢ Consider adding supplements to your regime. Do so judiciously.

➢ Try photobiomodulation therapy.

➢ Try cold therapy.

CHAPTER 4

STRESS:
Your Body's Physical, Mental, or Emotional Reaction to Pressure

STRESS CAN MAKE YOU SICK. When we worry, or are in a state of fear, our body has a physiological response which, when prolonged, makes us more vulnerable to disease. Chronic stress is one of the major contributors to dysfunction and disease. It is known to reactivate dormant viruses in your body. You can master all of the foundational pillars of health (nutrition, sleep, exercise), but if you are chronically stressed, your health will be adversely affected, and you won't feel well. It is estimated that 90 percent of doctor visits are due to illnesses related to stress. The main metrics used to measure stress include HRV (heart rate variability), blood pressure, cortisol, oxidative stress, and genetic factors.

LIFE IS 10 PERCENT WHAT HAPPENS TO YOU AND 90 PERCENT HOW YOU REACT

Stress can be physical, emotional, chemical, or microbial. The impact of chemical and microbial stress is discussed in chapter 5. While stress is unavoidable, it is modifiable. It is defined as the perception of a real or imagined event that can cause you harm. Your body has the same physiological response whether you are being chased by a tiger, you are worried that your kids are unsafe, or you believe (imaginarily or not) that your spouse is unfaithful. In all these examples, you are focused on things out of your control. Other triggers of stress include a bad diet, financial security, relationships, lack of downtime, regular deadlines, and even traffic-filled commutes. The ubiquitous existence of smartphones contributes to our stress. We are all always using our phones and losing important moments of presence. While we wait in line or have one minute to spare, our default response has become to do something on our phone whether it's to read and respond to emails and texts or to scroll through social media and the internet. Our brain needs downtime to solve problems. When showering, one can accomplish a lot of good thinking and problem-solving.

There are, of course, terrible experiences in life, such as the loss of a loved one, which triggers both grief and stress. The expression that life is 10 percent what happens to you and 90 percent how you react has great merit. It is thought that stress itself is not so bad, but rather it is one's perception of the stressful event. Stress management includes reframing your emotional relationship with stress, embracing it, and perceiving it as not so harmful but just a part of life.

THE BIOLOGY OF STRESS

Stress affects four major systems: the digestive system, immune system, nervous system, and hormonal system. When we perceive something stressful is about to occur, the amygdala portion of our brain becomes hypervigilant to keep us safe. This would be useful if the threat is real and current, but it is harmful when the stressful event is perceived or ongoing. Our brain's autonomic nervous system manages the way we respond to and recover from stress. The autonomic nervous system regulates heart rate, digestion, respiratory rate, pupillary response, urination, and sexual arousal. It controls the sympathetic nervous system, known as the fight-or-flight system, and the parasympathetic nervous system, known as the rest-and-digest system. As the stress is perceived, cortisol is released, and blood sugar is increased and directed toward muscles so we can run away from the imaginary or symbolic tiger. This is an evolutionary adaptation and an instinct to deal with a stressful or dangerous situation. As one's heart rate increases and blood flow is directed to the muscles, the digestive and immune systems slow down.

The vagus nerve, the longest and most complex of the twelve cranial nerves composing the autonomic nervous system, runs all the way from the brain stem through the face, neck, heart, lungs, and into the abdomen. In Latin, the definition of vagus is "wandering," and it certainly wanders throughout our body. This remarkable nerve regulates your autonomic nervous system, which in turn controls your internal organs. It stimulates certain muscles in the heart that help slow the heart rate. It also allows the brain to monitor and receive information about bodily functions.

THE VAGUS NERVE

The biology of stress requires a discussion of the vagus nerve.

THE DANCE BETWEEN THE SYMPATHETIC AND PARASYMPATHETIC NERVOUS SYSTEM

When the vagus nerve is triggering the sympathetic nervous system, energy, blood pressure, heart rate, and breathing rate all increase as a stress response. When the vagus nerve is triggering the parasympathetic nervous system, alertness, blood pressure, and heart rate are all decreased so that calm, relaxation, and digestion can occur. There is a fascinating bidirectional communication always taking place between your brain and other organs courtesy of the vagus nerve. Whether you are on high alert or in a state of calm depends upon the information conveyed by the vagus nerve. The sympathetic nerve and the parasympathetic nerve are switching in dominance throughout the day. A healthy person has increased sympathetic nerve activity as they become active during the day, and it switches to allow an increase of parasympathetic nerve activity at night. When one is experiencing a great deal of stress, both physical and mental during the day, these nerves begin to function improperly. Sympathetic nerve activity dominance results in a weakened immune system. Deep breathing and slow exhaling can redirect vagal activity when necessary. Exhalations should last twice as long as inhalations to create calm. When one breathes consciously and engages their diaphragm, the belly expands which causes the body to relax, the heart rate to slow, and relaxation to occur.

MEDITATION AND STRESS REDUCTION

Another scientifically proven way to reduce and manage stress is meditation. Nearly twelve years ago, I attended a seminar about the scientific research around the benefits of meditation, well before mediation books, apps, practices, and proponents became as ubiquitous as they are today. The seminar was conducted by a cognitive neuroscientist and a Tibetan monk. The research that the neuroscientist, Amishi Jha, had conducted was based on pre-deployment soldiers. She recounted that it was voluntary among the soldiers as to whether they wanted to participate in the study. Those who chose to participate were taught how to meditate before they were shipped out to Afghanistan with the goal of teaching the soldiers to maintain attention while in stressful situations. The type of meditation taught to the soldiers was "mindfulness meditation." Mindfulness is defined as the ability to be aware and attentive in the present without emotional reactivity or volatility.[49] The soldiers learned how to focus on their breathing and to detach their minds from emotions and thoughts while still observing their emotions and thoughts. The method was tested by recording brain waves to determine if focus and awareness were increased and if the ability to manage and recover from stress could improve. The results of the study showed that, in fact, meditation promoted cognitive resilience, attention, and working memory when faced with stress. I recall Dr. Jha saying that the soldiers who had chosen not to participate in the study observed how well their fellow soldiers did when deployed, and, later, they asked to have the same training. She shared elaborate graphs indicating dramatic changes in neural pathways resulting from mindfulness meditation. Further confirmation of the benefit of this practice was succinctly described by US Army Major Victor Won, when in 2010, he said, "It would be more effective for soldiers to learn and train mindfulness prior to deployment. [...] It is through finding peace within and clarity (that you) see that you are not the thoughts or the emotions that bind you and take you away into suffering. [...] In the present, you have the power to make changes to the situations affecting you. [...] With mindfulness, you can choose to see things as they are and accept them as they are [...] and then work to improve the situation if possible."[50]

There is no shortage of different kinds of meditation practices. To name just a few, Zen meditation, mindfulness meditation, Transcendental Meditation, and Kundalini yoga meditation all share the goal of encouraging a focus on heightened awareness, slowed breathing, and increased acceptance.

TRANSCENDENTAL MEDITATION

Transcendental Meditation is one that I have tried. It was started in India in the 1950s by Maharishi Mahesh Yogi and is now practiced all over the world. It is to be practiced twice a day for twenty minutes each time while silently chanting a mantra. Certified teachers teach the method and give you your own mantra. I can't confirm if everyone's mantra is different or the same because you are admonished to not disclose your mantra. The health effects of this meditation have been studied for more than fifty years. Hundreds of peer-reviewed studies on the practice of TM have been conducted by major universities and research centers that concluded that stress and anxiety were greatly reduced by a consistent practice, along with decreased depression, reduced insomnia, improved cardiovascular health, improved neurological health, reduced metabolic syndrome, and even increased longevity.

MY STORY

In the interest of full disclosure, TM was not a game changer for me. I had heard many reports from others who claimed that TM or other types of meditation changed their life. That was not my experience. I committed to the practice, as it is called, 100 percent. For about one full year, I did my meditation twice a day for twenty minutes each time, as prescribed. After the first year, I meditated once a day for twenty minutes. By year three, after taking the rather involved and not-inexpensive training, I stopped meditating altogether. Currently, I just think about meditating all the time. I tell myself daily, I should really meditate today. I am not sure what my excuse is other than the fact that I try so many different lifestyle alterations that I become overwhelmed by all of them and find the need to prioritize. I found the process of meditating exceedingly difficult. When I took the enlightening symposium on meditation, the Tibetan monk would end each of the three days with a guided meditation for the entire group. I really wanted to benefit from the process but found it more frustrating than stress reducing. The symposium took place just after the Fukushima nuclear power plant disaster. The crisis was paramount in my mind. When the Tibetan monk guided us through our meditation and told us to imagine the ocean gently lapping onto the shore, all I could think about was the nuclear waste from Japan making its way to the shores of California. By the end of the meditation session, I was far more worked up than before starting! I share my experience for those of you who have had similar experiences with meditation and found it difficult to maintain a consistent practice. While I may not have experienced the unabashed bliss that many meditators claim, I also do not feel particularly downtrodden that I did not maintain a consistent meditation practice. I have found that using different breathing techniques has been helpful in my stress reduction.

INCREASED GREY MATTER

Some of the other studies on the benefits of meditation include a 2014 Harvard study that showed the increase in grey-matter density of the brain because of meditating.[51] The study took place over fifty-six days and involved twenty-seven minutes of meditating each day. The eight-week program of mindfulness meditation showed that the meditators experienced an increase in the size of their hippocampus, the part of the brain responsible for learning and memory, and a decrease in their amygdala, the part of the brain associated with anxiety and stress response. All of these results were seen on an MRI scan and gave a new understanding that actual changes in the structure of the brain explain why people feel better when practicing meditation. This is further confirmation of the relatively new discovery about the plasticity of the brain.

A 2014 study conducted at the UCLA Brain Mapping Center suggested that meditation preserves the brain's grey matter.[52] This study included fifty people who meditated and fifty people who did not. Both groups showed a loss of grey matter over time, but the degree of loss was greater among those who did not meditate. Each group had twenty-eight men and twenty-two women, ranging in age from twenty-four to seventy-seven, and the length of time of meditation practice ranged from four to forty-six years, with an average of twenty years spent meditating. While the causal connections were found to be not definitive due to a multitude of factors in play, it was concluded that meditation did reduce the risks of loss of grey brain matter.

POSITIVE THINKING

Another area of stress management that isn't completely definitive but shows promise is the area of positive thinking. Researchers believe that positive thoughts may confer benefits against the inflammatory damage of stress and that negative emotions can weaken one's immune system.[53, 54] Positive thinking can help build resiliency, which is critical for the ability to adapt to stressful situations. Researchers found that personality traits such as optimism and pessimism can influence your health. Optimistic people tend to think more positively which helps them cope with stress better than pessimistic people. Pessimists can alter their thought processes and learn to think more positively. I suppose that the corollary of this is that pessimists are rarely disappointed, but I'm not sure that's a compelling reason to encourage pessimism. This doesn't mean that you have to view everything as downright cheery. Life is not always cheery, but it is helpful to look for the good in everything. Even the direst situations usually have something positive about them. The loss of a loved one is beyond painful, but it can be helpful to focus on the positive aspects of the loved one's life and the happy experiences shared.

EXERCISE

Exercise is another great method of stress management. You don't want to overdo your exercise because then you will be creating internal stress, or oxidative stress, but a moderate and consistent routine can be enormously beneficial. I am also aware that practitioners of yoga have had great success in stress management, but I cannot attest to that personally.

PETS

I can attest to the wonderful benefits, both the stress relieving and sheer enjoyment, of pets. An interesting report published by a European team of researchers reviewed evidence from sixty-nine individual studies on human and animal interactions. While most of the studies involved dogs, a few involved birds, farm animals, and fish in an aquarium. The report concluded that, based on the evidence, these human and animal interactions reduce stress and anxiety and have overall positive health impacts.[55]

WHY ZEBRAS DON'T GET CANCER

Robert Sapolsky, a professor of biology and neurology at Stanford University and a leading researcher in stress, wrote a terrific book (among others) called *Why Zebras Don't Get Ulcers*. The premise of the book is distinguishing between wild animals which frequently face life-threatening experiences and humans facing stress. When the zebra or other wild animal is being chased by a predator, the stress is episodic or fleeting. However, the stress which humans experience tends to be ongoing and chronic. Sapolsky explains how chronic stress can cause diseases like depression, ulcers, digestive issues, heart disease, insulin resistance, weight gain, fatigue, cognitive issues, and a weakened immune system.

HORMESIS

A related concept that I find fascinating is the concept of hormesis.

There are many examples of this phenomenon such as exposure to low doses of radiation, low doses of toxins, moderate exercise, and fasting or brief periods of no food. This is called a biphasic response because the response is dose dependent. The mechanism of utility here is that small doses of a bad thing can stimulate an adaptive response in our body and increase our resistance. This could have an application to the perceived threats that cause stress if we were able to recover quickly and not have a prolonged experience. Perhaps if we could move on quickly and shake it off, we could develop greater resistance.

Hormesis is a biological phenomenon where one has the opposite response to a particular kind of stressor depending upon the dose. These stressors are different from the unrelenting stress we face daily, but the concept sheds light on our biological response. When we are exposed to a stressor that is harmful at a moderate or higher dose, the same stressor at a low dose can be beneficial.

MEASURING STRESS

It is useful to track your stress levels. There is an expression that says, you can't manage what you can't measure. Collecting quantitative data is the first step to optimizing your health because you know specifically what to focus on and the results of your efforts. One effective way to measure your stress level is to test your heart rate variability, or HRV. The rhythm of a healthy heart is, contrary to what one might think, irregular. The interval between consecutive heartbeats is constantly changing. When you measure your HRV, you get an assessment of the balance between your sympathetic nervous system and your parasympathetic nervous system. It reveals how you cope with stress and your level of resilience. The lower your HRV number is, the more compromised your nervous system. A low number can also be an indication that you haven't recovered from a previous day's workout and that you may be overexercising and need a day off to rest and recover. Ideally, you want a high degree of variability which indicates flexibility and the ability to adapt to stress. Breathing, fitness, thoughts, and emotions all impact your autonomic nervous system and, therefore, your HRV. The way in which you can track your HRV is through either an HRV-tracking watch strap called WHOOP or an Ōura Ring. These devices connect to apps on your phone and give you a wealth of terrific information. Other stress measuring devices include those made by Polar, Garmin, HeartMath, Lief, and Biostrap.

GENETICS AND STRESS

The relationship between genes and the susceptibility to stress, anxiety, depression, and other mood disorders is not definitive. Some experts think there is no connection while others are certain that genetics inform our body's response to stress. David Goldman, MD, chief of the NIAAA (National Institute on Alcohol Abuse and Alcoholism) has identified gene variants that affect the expression of a signaling molecule called neuropeptide Y (NPY). Goldman explains: "Found in brain and many other tissues, NPY regulates diverse functions, including appetite, weight, and emotional responses." He concludes that genetic factors play an important role in mood and anxiety disorder.[56]

SPECIFIC STRESS-RELATED GENES

The following are genes that have been identified to have a connection to stress:

OXTR gene: This gene is associated with reduced oxytocin signaling, which may result in increased anxiety.

GABRA6 gene: This gene may impair GABA function and has been associated with higher anxiety.

SLC6A4 gene: This gene is responsible for transporting serotonin in your brain. It is thought to impact your levels of stress and happiness.

HCRTR1 gene: This gene may predispose you to a higher likelihood of anxiety.

CNR1 gene: This gene also may predispose you to a higher likelihood of anxiety.

SOD2 gene: This gene helps protect the body from oxidative stress. The higher the activity with this gene, the greater the protection against neurodegenerative disease.

Klotho gene: This gene is known as the "longevity gene." High activity of this gene is associated with reduced oxidative stress and inflammation. There are many variants of the klotho gene and several are correlated with a positive impact on cholesterol, blood pressure, stroke, and other life-shortening issues.

Chronic stress affects every organ in your body. It shrinks the hippocampus, the memory center in your brain, and decreases your resistance to disease. Since living in today's world makes it impossible to avoid stress, it is essential to learn how to manage your response to stress.

Usually, we all highly over-estimate the dangers in our life, so we need to learn to change our interpretation of a stressful event. Our response is wholly dependent on the meaning we assign to the stressful incident. The goal must be to reduce anxiety and stress to strengthen your immune system, optimize your health, and improve the overall quality of your life.

ACTION STEPS

➢ Prioritize stress reduction.

➢ Experiment with different meditation practices.

➢ Try different breathing techniques.

➢ Invest in a device to measure your HRV.

➢ Reframe your perspective and response to stressful events.

CHAPTER 5

TOXINS:
Deny These Insidious Invaders

THE US PERMITS OVER EIGHTY-FIVE thousand chemicals to be used in our food supply, water, and commercial materials. Most of these have not been tested for safety. Increasing evidence indicates that exposure to the ubiquitous presence of toxins is a big factor in the rise of chronic disease.

It was believed that the placenta protected the cord blood and the fetus from toxic chemical exposure for years. We now know that this is untrue. Based on the Environmental Working Group (EWG) studies, newborn babies have over two hundred environmental toxins in their umbilical cord blood. The studies investigated industrial chemicals, pollutants, and pesticides in umbilical cord blood. Specifically, the EWG found hydrocarbons, dioxins, furans, pesticides, flame retardants, industrial lubricants, plastics, lead, mercury, PFCs, and many other toxicants.[57]

The United States is the largest global producer of chemicals, introducing two thousand new chemicals each year. The federal law governing these chemicals was established in 1976 and is called the Toxic Substances Control Act (TSCA). It took forty years for this rather insubstantial regulation to be updated. In 2016, a new law was passed requiring the Environmental Protection Agency

(EPA) to determine "unreasonable risk of injury to health and the environment."[58]

CHEMICAL COMBINATIONS

In the past, the focus on whatever meager testing took place was on looking at one chemical at a time without considering the risk of exposure to combinations of chemicals. It is now known and accepted that there is a definite synergistic effect of exposure to chemical combinations, like the increased risk for toxic interactions when combining multiple pharmaceutical medications instead of taking just one at a time. Combinations of chemicals present a greater risk than even singular chemical exposure.

CHEMICAL EXPOSURE AND DISEASE

The reality is that hundreds of clinical studies disprove this claim as they track individuals and the clear association between chemical exposure and disease. The following describes what I perceive to be some of the worst chemicals we are exposed to in our consumer products.

Another deficiency in the regulations of chemicals is that it takes approximately seven years to review each chemical. Then, the law gives the manufacturer an additional five years to remedy whatever problem is found. Therefore, we allow a minimum of twelve years for each potentially harmful chemical to remain lurking in our environment. The CDC and the manufacturers of these chemicals defend their position with the assertion that the "mere presence of a chemical" does not prove harm.

By no means is this a complete list. I strongly suggest searching the internet for additional harmful chemicals to avoid.

ACRYLAMIDE

This chemical has been classified as a "possible carcinogen." It is used in several industries such as paper, construction, textiles, cosmetics, food processing and food packaging, plastics, and in treating drinking water and wastewater. This chemical can also occur naturally in foods such as French fries, potato chips, cereal, and grain-based food from a chemical reaction after high-temperature cooking.

PHTHALATES

These are an entire family of petroleum-based chemicals. They are used to make plastic and polyvinyl chloride (PVC) soft and flexible. We find them in personal care products, wood finishes, detergents, solvents, insecticides, building materials, meat and dairy products, and fast food. The FDA has banned some of these chemicals from children's toys and teething products. A 2003 study in *Environmental Health Perspectives*[59] suggested that phthalates can alter DNA integrity in human sperm. Another study, conducted in 2004 at the Harvard School of Public Health, pointed out that the coating of medications often is coated in a substance containing phthalates.[60] Although phthalates are widely considered endocrine-disrupting chemicals (EDCs) and have been banned from cosmetics made in the European Union, the FDA and the American Chemistry Council have stated that phthalates do not pose a risk to human health. It is staggering how much conflicting evidence exists about these materials.

The show *60 Minutes* did an exposé on these chemicals and referenced studies linking phthalates to diabetes, asthma, and male reproduction. One such study, "The Association between Asthma and Allergic Symptoms in Children and Phthalates in House Dust," by Carl-Gustaf Bornehag et al. confirms that there is cause for concern. [61,62]

TRICLOSAN

Triclosan is an antibacterial and antifungal agent used in a wide range of consumer products. These include toothpaste, soap, deodorants, skincare products, detergents, cleaning products, toys, kitchenware, and even athletic clothing and food packaging. Because most of these end up washed down the drain, the chemical ends up in our oceans and other waterways and has been found in fish that we eat. As of 2017, the FDA has banned the marketing of soap and antiseptic washes containing triclosan in the US. The European Union has gone further and has banned triclosan from all personal care products. In the US, for some unknown reason, we still allow triclosan to be used in toothpaste. A biochemist from the University of Maine, Julie Gosse, PhD, has published studies on the harmful effects of triclosan on one's mitochondria.[63] A spokesperson from a company that still makes the toothpaste with the toxin countered Gosse's study with the assertion that "mice metabolize triclosan far differently than humans [...]." While mice are not humans, they are the test subjects for most chemicals. While their metabolisms may function differently from humans, there is still great cause for concern when using a triclosan product. I suggest that those who are interested check the website beyondpesticides.org for a list of triclosan products.

A friend of mine was experiencing severe and uncomfortable canker sores in her mouth. She was advised to switch kinds of toothpaste to a nontoxic brand. As soon as she did this, her canker sores went away and never returned.

BPA (BISPHENOL A) AND BPS (BISPHENOL S)

In 2015, Senator Dianne Feinstein (D-California) introduced a bill to eliminate BPA, an industrial chemical that had found its way into many consumer products. You find the chemical in currency, cans, paper receipts, Tupperware, plastic wrap, and plastic water bottles, to name just a few consumer products. It was replaced by a different chemical substance called bisphenol S (BPS), which is apparently worse or more harmful than its predecessor. This bait-and-switch act is like the additives used to replace lead in gasoline. These actions represent compliance with regulations but end up causing more harm than the original banned substance. Similarly, and quite noteworthy, the chemicals that cities put into the water supply to kill microbes are far worse than the microbes!

TITANIUM DIOXIDE

While this is a naturally occurring material, it has been classified as a Group 2 carcinogen by the International Agency for Research on Cancer (IARC). In the US, it currently has the designation of GRAS, generally recognized as safe, but, reading between the lines, I get a distinct impression that this means, "We don't really know how safe this is." Titanium dioxide is a pigment used to enhance whiteness in a variety of products, including food, creamer, candy, toothpaste, chewing gum, sunscreen, bronzers, foundations, concealers, soaps, diaper creams, lotions, and even some medications and supplements. There is a different variation of titanium dioxide used in paints, plastics, and paper products. Scientists base toxicity concerns around topical exposure, digestive system exposure, and respiratory exposure.

Animal studies have linked inhalation of titanium dioxide to lung tumor development. Since titanium dioxide tends to be only partially pure, it can be contaminated with lead, arsenic, and mercury. It is noteworthy that Dunkin' recently stopped the use of titanium dioxide out of concern for the potential of toxicity. The potential hazards are largely due to the nanoparticles (microscopic particles) of titanium dioxide and their potential to cause oxidative stress resulting in cell damage, cell death, and increased inflammation.[64]

Another research paper focused on titanium dioxide nanoparticles confirms the dangers of this additive.[65] While additional research is needed on titanium dioxide, I believe that you will be better off if you can find alternative products without it. If possible, avoid it.

PARABENS

These are a group of chemicals that are preservatives used in cosmetic and pharmaceutical products. They are used to prevent the growth of bacteria and mold and extend these products' shelf life. The prominent names to familiarize yourself with are methylparaben, ethylparaben, butylparaben, isobutylparaben, and propylparaben. The FDA does not regulate the use of these chemicals, and they don't appear to be concerned about them. Tap into the EWG's Skin Deep cosmetics database which lists chemicals found in personal care products that one should avoid.[66] This website references multiple studies about the hazards of parabens. Most of the studies referenced illustrate male and female reproductive harm and increased risk of cancer from the use of products containing parabens.

The studies also document that parabens are xenoestrogens in that they mimic estrogen and can cause hormonal imbalance and an increased risk of breast cancer.

As an additional message of caution, several companies state that their products are "paraben-free." Still, they have simply substituted the suspect chemical with other synthetic substances that may be just as or even more harmful.

OTHER HARMFUL CHEMICAL INGREDIENTS

Any product, including personal care products, laundry products, perfumes, candles, and anything else containing the word "fragrance," is toxic. Unless essential oils are used to provide the fragrance, toxic synthetic chemicals should be avoided. When trying to reduce one's toxic load, it is best to choose "fragrance-free" products.

Sodium lauryl sulfate (SLS) and sodium laureth sulfate are chemicals known as surfactants and are found in shampoo, toothpaste, mouthwash, soap, and bodywash. Studies have linked SLS to cancer, neurotoxicity, organ toxicity, skin irritation, and endocrine disruption.

Other ingredients to look for and to avoid in your products are diethanolamine (DEA), triethanolamine (TEA) and monoethanolamine (MEA), chromium, dioxane, xylenol, oleth, ceteareth, PEG, methylisothiazolinone (MIT), hydroquinone, dimethicone, methicone, cyclomethicone, triclosan, coal tar, propylene glycol, acrylamide, and all chemical colors with numbers.

Another category of petroleum-based products or petrochemicals that you should avoid include petroleum jelly, mineral oil, paraffin wax, toluene, benzene, petrolatum, BHA, BHT, and butanol or butyl. These are in perfume, hair dye, lotion, cosmetics, deodorant, toothpaste, vanilla ice cream (artificial flavoring), preservatives, vitamins and capsules, pain relievers, plastic bags, clothing, detergent, and golf balls. When buying sunscreen, try to buy one that doesn't contain oxybenzone or octinoxate. Both chemicals have been shown to cause biochemical or cellular changes and endocrine disruption.

The FDA defines natural flavors as anything derived from something that originated in nature. This is without regard to how these "natural flavors" get processed before inclusion into your food. According to the EWG, natural flavors can consist of fifty to one hundred different components.

The term "natural flavors" seems to describe innocuous ingredients that might even be healthy. But that is not the case.

They can include glycerin, corn syrup, solvents, emulsifiers, and preservatives. These are all a far cry from nature! Be wary!

XENOESTROGENS

These synthetic or chemical compounds mimic the effect of estrogen. Their molecular structure is close enough to estrogen that they can bind to the estrogen receptor. This results in the interference with your ability to excrete estrogen and leads to estrogen dominance and alters your hormones' normal functions. Exposure to these endocrine disrupters is through contaminated food and liquids, absorption of consumer products through the skin and mucous membranes, and through inhalation. Some of the chemicals called xenoestrogens include parabens, benzophenone, 4-methylbenzylidene camphor, BPA, phthalates, polybrominated diphenyl ethers (PBDEs), and polychlorinated biphenyls (PCBs).

You will find these chemicals in sunscreen, plastic products, building materials, furnishings, electronics, cars, food coloring, food preservatives, artificial food additives, paints, adhesives, lubricants, electrical oils, commercially raised meat and dairy, tap water, pesticides, herbicides, fungicides, cleaning products, canned goods, cash register receipts, air fresheners, laundry products, cosmetics, shampoo, nail polish and remover, deodorant, body lotion, fragrance, and chlorine and chlorine byproducts. The conditions which have been connected to exposure to xenoestrogens include cancer, infertility, obesity, diabetes, and thyroid disruption.

HEAVY METALS

While these wreak absolute havoc on your body, they occur naturally and occur in many places you would not expect. The worst of the bunch include aluminum arsenide, cadmium, lead, and mercury.

While aluminum is not considered the worst of heavy metals, it is a matter of the dose. Excessive doses are known to be harmful. Despite many of these toxins being banned in Europe, Canada, and Japan, the US merely limits their usage.

ALUMINUM

Aluminum is the most plentiful metal on earth. Low levels of aluminum exposure tend not to be harmful. Once again, it is the dose that causes toxicity. Exposure is through air, food, and water. Many household items contain aluminum, as do vaccines, medications, paint, fuel additives, deodorants, cookware, food additives, containers, shampoo, and cosmetics. Some of the adverse outcomes from aluminum toxicity include lung issues, nervous system issues, bone disease, brain disease, anemia, and impaired iron absorption. One's lymph system and thyroid gland have both been found to be adversely affected by aluminum toxicity. A mystifying increase in thyroid disease in the general population does not seem to be getting sufficient attention. People with impaired kidney function are at the highest risk of aluminum toxicity because they have an impaired ability to excrete aluminum.

An interesting study about aluminum toxicity concluded that exposure to aluminum may result in mitochondrial dysfunction and lead to oxidative stress.[67]

ARSENIC

Arsenic is in the air, water supply, soil, and food supply. According to articles published in *Environmental Health Perspective* and PubMed, high levels have been detected in foods like brown rice, chickens, eggs, and the water supply.[68,69] Other studies show a link between arsenic and an increase in type 2 diabetes, cerebrovascular disease, cancer, liver disease, lung issues, and skin lesions.[70] This element is difficult to avoid entirely because of its ubiquitous nature. The association with serious disease appears to be a result of consistent, long-term exposure.

CADMIUM

Cadmium is another naturally occurring toxic metal used largely in agriculture and manufacturing that is also found in batteries, smoke, car exhaust, certain meats, and seafood. This metal's adverse effects include cardiovascular, renal, gastrointestinal, neurological, repro-ductive, and respiratory issues. It is also known to be estrogenic and has been linked to different types of cancer.

LEAD

Yet one more naturally occurring heavy metal, lead, has dangerous toxic effects. Children are particularly vulnerable to the damaging effects of lead, but adults can have a great deal of lead accumulation and attendant problems. In 1978, the US federal government banned lead-based paint, and some states banned it even earlier. Lead in gasoline was slowly phased out, and by January 1, 1996, the Clean Air Act banned leaded gasoline for use in new vehicles other than aircraft, racing cars, farm equipment, and marine engines. Lead still exists in the air, water, food, and some consumer products.

MERCURY

More than a decade ago, the news was filled with actor Jeremy Piven's story of suffering from debilitating illnesses from excessive sushi and Chinese herb consumption. After consuming sushi twice daily over an extended period, Piven experienced dizziness and severe, unrelenting fatigue. He went through extensive testing, all unable to reveal the source of his discomfort. It wasn't until he found a doc-tor who thought to test Piven's heavy-metal-toxicity levels that he learned that his mercury levels were almost six times the upper limit of normal and allowable. Part of the reason that it was so difficult for

Piven to get a proper diagnosis is that blood tests only show recent toxin exposure. Frequent and consistent toxin exposure hides in your tissues and does not always show up in your blood work.

Symptoms of mercury poisoning include muscle weakness, peripheral neuropathy resulting from nerve damage (this is a numbness and burning sensation in hands and feet), issues with vision and coordination, and

> Mercury is released into the air in huge quantities through pollution. It becomes methylmercury and lands in oceans, streams, other waterways, and soil. The fish containing the highest levels of methylmercury are king mackerel, swordfish, tuna, marlin, halibut, and shark.

problems with neuromuscular function, such as difficulty in raising one's arms and legs. If not treated properly, mercury poisoning can result in cardiac arrest, kidney failure, and even psychiatric problems.

Additional sources of these dangerous metals include broken fluorescent light bulbs, amalgams, thimerosal in vaccines, cosmetics, food, cleaning products, dental care products, hair care products, sunscreen, eye drops, cookware, paint, carpet, and laundry products.

When humans ingest and absorb high levels of mercury, it binds to any tissue and can trigger a cytokine attack. If your gut is healthy, you are less likely to absorb harmful quantities of mercury. Mercury is the most highly neurotoxic element and is also immunotoxic. It is even toxic to the digestive system, our bones, and the thyroid gland. It is becoming apparent that there is a relationship between mercury exposure and Alzheimer's disease.[71] Other studies confirm that mercury hides in adipose tissue and explain why the detoxification process can be difficult.[72]

In Japan, methylmercury poisoning causes a disease named Minamata disease due to people eating fish tainted with methylmercury found in water that was near a chemical plant.

The number of stories of individual experiences with mercury poisoning is so plentiful that there is a website devoted exclusively to this topic. It is www.mercurystories.com.

TYPES OF TOXINS

Toxins are classified in different ways. Sometimes, they are organized according to chemical (both inorganic and organic compounds); sometimes they are classified as biological toxins, which are toxic compounds secreted by an organism; other times they are divided into endotoxins, made inside of the body, and exotoxins, entering the body from the environment. However they are classified, it is important to understand that different toxins affect different organs. Neurotoxins affect the brain, hepatotoxins affect the liver, nephrotoxins affect the kidneys, and dermatoxins affect the skin.

ENDOTOXINS

Endotoxins are produced within the body and are usually lipopolysaccharides (LPS). These are toxic chemicals that inflame the gut, resulting in a leaky gut, attack the immune system, and increase your overall toxic burden. Examples of these negative pathogenic bacteria that can wreak havoc on your health are *Escherichia coli*, *salmonella, shigella, pseudomonas, Neisseria, Haemophilus influenzae*, and *Vibrio cholerae*. Endotoxins often influence both obesity and type 2 diabetes, conditions that plague Americans.

EXOTOXINS

Exotoxins are even more toxic than endotoxins. Only a tiny number of exotoxins are necessary to cause toxicity. These are produced by both gram-negative and gram-positive bacteria. Examples of these nasty organisms include cholera, tetanus, botulism, and that particularly frightening, flesh-eating bacteria such as group A strep or staph.

MYCOTOXINS

These toxins are derived from mold and fungus and cause DNA damage. They break down myelin, which are the fatty sheaths that insulate your neurons and allow them to send information throughout your brain. The breakdown of myelin is a primary component of multiple sclerosis, Parkinson's disease, and Alzheimer's disease. There is a startling study that revealed the findings of fungal infections inside the neurons of Alzheimer's patients.[73]

EXPOSOME

In 2005, epidemiologist Dr. Christopher Wild developed the concept called "exposome" to describe the total exposure of all environmental toxins one experiences beginning at conception and throughout life. These include pollutants, toxins, nutrition, stress, and lifestyle and represent the non-genetic factors that affect your health. The real issue is the cumulation of exposure over a lifetime. A small dose or brief exposure triggers an inflammatory response. While we may not sense this muted response at first, if regulators do not remove more toxins from the supply chain, the continuous exposure over years and decades sets the stage for disease. Included among the myriad of ills that toxins present to your health are extreme damage caused to mitochondria, damage to your DNA, damage to organs, and the displacement of minerals.

DETOXIFICATION

The human body is designed brilliantly to detoxify through different physiological mechanisms. If we weren't able to detoxify, we would die. The main detoxification organs are the liver, the colon, the kidneys, the lungs, and the skin. When the body recognizes foreign substances that are toxic, its detoxification pathways aid in the excretion and elimination of these substances.

TWO PHASES OF DETOXIFICATION

The body uses two phases of detoxification, referred to as phase one detox and phase two detox. In phase one, enzymes called cytochrome P450 are responsible for the breakdown of toxins through oxidation, reduction, and hydrolysis. An area of concern in this phase is the creation of free radicals during the process. The best way to avoid that is to reduce toxin exposure. The next phase, phase two, is referred to as *conjugation,* and its function is to make the toxins less reactive and to convert them into a water-soluble form so they can be excreted more effectively. The process begins in the liver as it filters out the substances from entering your bloodstream and moves them onto the gall bladder and kidneys. The kidneys continue the filtration process and excrete the toxins in your urine. The gallbladder, along with the production of bile, eliminates toxins through a bowel movement. The colon or the digestive system is filled with both good and bad bacteria. One of the colon's main functions is to excrete waste through bowel movements to prevent harmful substances from accumulating.

The lungs filter out the toxins such as fumes, allergens, mold, and other airborne toxins that enter your body while breathing. The skin, our largest organ, facilitates the excretion of toxins through sweat. The fat-soluble toxins are broken down into fat and converted into water-soluble substances to be excreted as fluid. The most effective means of toxin elimination are through bowel movements, urine, and sweat.

The ability to detoxify effectively depends on the health, age, and genetics of the individual. Certain genetic variations, as well as nutritional deficiencies, are known to interfere with effective detoxification. When the detoxification pathways are blocked or not working correctly to facilitate elimination, the toxins can be reabsorbed and recirculated. Sometimes this occurs when attempts to detoxify using certain supplements neglect to include the appropriate binders. These binders are critical to prevent the toxins released from the tissues into the bloodstream from becoming reabsorbed. Some of the symptoms of toxic reabsorption include fatigue, headaches, skin issues, and many others.

ANNE'S STORY

My friend Anne is an example of what can go wrong when attempting to detoxify by oneself or under an inexperienced health-care provider's guidance. Anne was experiencing an unexplained malaise which included muscle weakness, tingling in her feet and hands, and even changes in her vision. Her neighbor referred her to a doctor who suggested that she go through a "chelation process." Unfortunately for Anne, this doctor was inexperienced, didn't understand the implications of this process, and administered it incorrectly.

My friend was left feeling even worse than she had before beginning the chelation. She had two years of extreme fatigue, headaches, and gut issues in addition to her previous issues. This cautionary tale is a reminder to always consult with experienced providers and ask many questions.

The doctor neglected to add critical binders to the protocol, allowing the removed toxins and heavy metals to recirculate and reabsorb into Anne's system. Binders are like little sponges which attach to the toxins making them easier to eliminate from your body. Two examples of binders are activated charcoal and pyrophyllite clay. When binders are not used, the process of detox involves your liver processing the toxins, your intestines reabsorbing the toxins, and then your liver recirculating the toxins again.

MTHFR GENETIC VARIATION AND DETOXIFICATION

An example of a genetic variation affecting one's detoxification efficacy is methylenetetrahydrofolate reductase (MTHFR). This hard-to-pronounce enzyme converts folate to its active form, L-methylfolate, and is critical to methylation. Methylation has many functions, including DNA repair, DNA synthesis, tissue and cell regeneration, amino acid balance, immune system function, inflammation regulation, and liver function.

Specifically, this gene increases sulfation for the excretion of heavy metals and the excretion of environmental toxins and pathogens out of the body. I know that this all sounds complicated, but it's essential to know that methylation and its dysfunction have been implicated in hundreds of medical conditions. Methylation affects your detoxification ability. If you can't detoxify efficiently, you are at a higher risk for vitamin B deficiency, Alzheimer's disease, cardiovascular disease, stroke, gastrointestinal issues, anxiety, depression, autoimmune disease, and cancer. I hope I haven't alarmed you too much with this information. The reality is that 30–50 percent of the population may be affected by this genetic variation. If you test positive for it (as I have), it is not a guarantee that you will develop a disease but means that you are at a higher risk for certain diseases. As with nearly every risk, there are mitigating factors that you can adopt. These include the same ones we keep hearing about which are sleep, stress reduction, and nutrition. When relying on nutrition to mitigate the risks of poor methylation, you can eat foods like broccoli, lentils and beans, avocados, leafy greens, and fruits. Some herbs and supplements are thought to improve methylation, offset MTHFR genetic variation, and help with detoxification. Consult a skilled practitioner if you want to use supplements.

In 1986, the state of California acknowledged the need to regulate the toxic chemicals that were causing harm and passed Proposition 65, also known as the Safe Drinking Water and Toxic Enforcement Act.[74] While it could use some updating as to the types of damage which must be avoided, this act has improved public awareness of the environmental toxins we regularly face. The act requires a warning label placed on all consumer products and locations which contain chemicals known to cause cancer or reproductive harm. It states, "known to the State of California to cause [cancer] [birth defects or other reproductive harm]."

The law is politically controversial because it places the burden on the companies to incur the costs associated with testing products, developing less harmful alternatives if necessary, and providing a warning on their products. The controversy is due in part to the fact that the law has resulted in a large payday for plaintiffs' attorneys, as anyone can sue over a product missing the warning. In 2014, Governor Jerry Brown called for the law to be reformed.

It is impossible now to eliminate all toxic exposure. It is, however, possible to make substantial reductions. The following recommendations illustrate a number of ways you can lower your toxic burden.

FOOD

If your budget allows, try to eat organic whenever possible. Websites such as Pesticide Action Network and the EPA website can inform you of the most egregious pesticides. Farmers spray certain foods such as nuts, coffee, and tea with huge quantities of pesticides because they are vulnerable to pests. Packaged foods are chock-full of preservatives like artificial coloring, MSG, sodium benzoate, sodium nitrate, nitrite, and bromate. If you can replace packaged and processed foods with fresh foods, you will reduce your chemical load. If you choose to eat animal products, select products that are raised without antibiotics and hormones.

I hate to be the bearer of bad news, but for the wine and beer lovers out there, there is a lot of glyphosate (weed killer) in most wine and beer. A study published by the U.S. PIRG (U.S. Public Interest Research Group) discusses twenty brands of wine and beer that were evaluated for glyphosate.[75]

THE DIRTY DOZEN

This list compiled by the Environmental Working Group (EWG) is composed of the fruits and vegetables grown using the most pesticides and with the highest level of pesticide residue. The EWG gathered the data for these lists from the United States Department of Agriculture's Pesticide Data Program. The suggestion is that the following should be purchased only when organic options are available.

1. Strawberries
2. Spinach
3. Kale
4. Nectarines
5. Apples
6. Grapes
7. Peaches
8. Cherries
9. Pears
10. Tomatoes
11. Celery
12. Potatoes

THE CLEAN FIFTEEN

This list, also published by the EWG, shows the fruits and vegetables with the lowest amount of pesticide residue.

1. Avocado
2. Sweet Corn
3. Pineapple
4. Onion
5. Papaya
6. Sweet Peas (Frozen)
7. Eggplant

8. Asparagus

9. Cauliflower

10. Cantaloupe

11. Broccoli

12. Mushrooms

13. Cabbage

14. Honeydew Melon

15. Kiwi

WATER

While the federal Safe Drinking Water Act resulted in much safer water, there are still plenty of contaminants and pollutants in our water supply.

Even bottled water is known to contain industrial chemicals and bacteria, so the best bet is filtered water. There is a broad range of water filters depending upon your budget, and any filter is better than no filter, but a reverse-osmosis filter is the only way to get rid of arsenic in your water supply. If you can, you want to consider filters for both your kitchens and showers. Choosing a water filter involves substantial research. Many different water filtration processes exist, ranging from distillation to reverse osmosis, and even more companies that manufacture these all-important additions to your life. If you have a plastic shower curtain, you run the risk of phthalate release when hot water runs on the shower curtain. Consider replacing it with a nonplastic curtain.

The EWG has identified more than 280 contaminants found in US tap water. If you can avoid tap water, you can minimize your ingestion of pesticides, fertilizers, pharmaceuticals, industrial solvents, and other harmful chemicals.

AIR

An air filter, or air purifier, is an excellent investment for cleaning toxins and particulates from the air inside your home. Indoor air quality, particularly in office buildings where windows do not open, can present many problems. Even gyms have tainted air due to the carpet releasing VOCs (volatile organic compounds), the ubiquitous presence of mold, and the harsh, chemical-laden cleaning fluids used. It is not always possible or practical to exercise outdoors, but when it is, choose to do that! If I can stress one thing regarding air, it would be the total and complete avoidance of using air fresheners. They do not freshen the air at all but instead mask the air with a synthetic soup of dangerous and disgusting chemicals. If you are desirous of scenting your air, use a diffuser or a candle made with essential oils (if they don't contain terpenes and are devoid of nasty chemicals). Another way to clean the inside air is using certain plants that naturally remove harmful chemicals. NASA has identified a list of these air-filtering plants. The list can be found in chapter 19.

You have many options for high-efficiency machines when choosing an air purifier for your home or office. The brands vary according to price and the size and number of particles the filters/purifiers can capture. There are several ratings, but two critical ratings are MPR, the Microparticle Performance Rating, and MERV, the Minimum Efficiency Reporting Value. Also of note is the HEPA (high-efficiency particulate air) standard, which requires that an air filter remove at least 99.97 percent of microparticles. A list of dependable brands of air purifiers can be found in chapter 19.

COOKWARE AND KITCHENWARE

Nonstick cookware, while much easier to clean, contains harmful synthetic chemicals called PFASs (per- and polyfluoroalkyl substances). These substances leach into the food while cooking. These chemicals exist in stain-, heat-, and water-resistant products as well as cookware. Several terrific companies are manufacturing non-toxic cookware. You can reduce your exposure to many offending chemicals using stainless steel, glass, cast iron, or ceramic cookware. Other ways to reduce chemicals while cooking include using a bamboo steamer for cooking vegetables and using tools made from ceramic, wood, stainless steel, or bamboo. It is also good to transfer nuts, seeds, and beans from their plastic package into reusable glass containers. Avoid using plastic or synthetic cutting boards and only use those made from wood. Instead of plastic wrap, use silicone lids, glass containers, Stasher bags made from silicone, or beeswax wrap. Don't buy eggs in Styrofoam cartons—or hot coffee, for that matter. Styrofoam is really bad news! Glass bottles are preferable to plastic for drinking and condiments. Instead of aluminum foil, unbleached, chlorine-free parchment paper will be a good substitute. A list of nontoxic cookware brands can be found in chapter 19.

CLEANING PRODUCTS

There are terrific nontoxic alternatives to sprays, cleaners, detergents, soaps, sponges, and mops that fill most of our homes. Conventional products are filled with toxic ingredients like bleach, silica, nonyl-phenol ethoxylates, 2-butoxyethanol, 2-hexoxyethanol, formalde-hyde, and APEs (alkylphenol ethoxylates). When you are purchasing cleaning products, look for these ingredients and avoid the product! There are plenty of do-it-yourself formulas on the internet to replace these toxic products. One alternative is to use distilled white vinegar combined with water as a cleaning fluid. If you are not inclined to do it yourself, several wonderful brands have a low or zero toxin exposure. Some of these brands can be found in chapter 19.

PERSONAL CARE PRODUCTS

This category is quite broad and covers makeup, perfume, tooth-paste, mouthwash, dental floss, nail polish, deodorant, shampoo, conditioner, hair color, bodywash, shaving cream, skin cleanser, and moisturizer. The ingredients to look for and to avoid include resor-cinol, coumarin (used to kill rodents), p-aminophenol, propane, butane, isobutane (used as an aerosol propellant), aluminum, diox-ins, lead, parabens, phthalates, sodium fluoride, PFCs, and ethox-ylated ingredients. Often, this group of products is contaminated and toxic. Lipstick contains twenty to forty ingredients (too many to put on such a small item) and often contains lead, mercury, cad-mium, and arsenic. Petroleum is another common ingredient found in these products and contains contaminants that are carcinogenic and endocrine disruptors. The ECHA (European Chemicals Agency) website is a good source. While products in the US are not required to comply with these regulations, it is a great reference. Some com-panies that produce nontoxic products can be found in chapter 19.

MATTRESSES AND BEDDING

Think of how much time we all spend in bed. Many states have enacted laws requiring mattresses to contain fire retardants to pre-vent smoking-in-bed deaths. As a result, we spend hours every night absorbing and inhaling the chemicals from the fire retardants and the content of memory foam and other chemicals like petrochem-icals, polyurethane, polyvinyl chloride, formaldehyde, phthalates, and boric acid. This concern applies to pillows as well, and there are many nontoxic alternatives available. Look for 100 percent natural materials like wool, cotton, hemp, bamboo, and natural latex. A few brands that are dependable and safe can be found in chapter 19.

PEST CONTROL

Most pesticides are carcinogenic, among other things. There are less toxic methods to rid your life of pests. Soapy water is a great solution to get rid of an ant invasion. Catnip supposedly repels cockroaches, diatomaceous earth can help with flea control, and if you sprinkle cayenne pepper, citrus oil on a rag, lemon juice, cinnamon, or coffee grounds, then many unwanted critters will go elsewhere.

If you are intrigued enough to research the toxins in your environment, there are many great resources: EWG, Think Dirty, whatsonmyfood.org, and CAS.org which is a chemical database.

Our environment has changed dramatically over the last 150 years. In many ways, it has improved, but there is a cost that accompanies improvements and advancements. There is a known association between toxic chemical exposure and chronic disease. The symptoms of this association are not always apparent at first. Because toxins accumulate and hide in our organs and adipose tissue (fat) and our brain, we must take serious steps to reduce our exposure.

My sincere hope for the future is that we conduct further research, implement greater education about the ways to lower toxin exposure, pass better environmental regulations, and fight for environmental justice. Lower socioeconomic circumstances must not allow for an increased risk of toxic exposure.

ACTION STEPS

➢ Eat organic food whenever possible.

➢ Minimize or eliminate your use of plastics. Replace with glass, ceramic, or stainless steel.

➢ Refer to the Dirty Dozen and Clean Fifteen on the EWG website and buy your produce accordingly.

➢ Filter your water.

➢ Filter your air. Invest in an air filter or air-filtering plants.

➢ Replace toxic cookware with nontoxic brands.

➢ Replace your toxic cleaning products with nontoxic brands or use white vinegar and water.

➢ Determine whether your personal care products are ladened with chemicals and harmful toxins.

➢ Invest in a nontoxic mattress.

➢ Stop using pesticides.

CHAPTER 6

SLEEP:
Your Critical Appointment
with the Sandman

IT IS ESTIMATED THAT 40 percent of Americans get inadequate sleep.[76]

LESLIE'S STORY

My friend Leslie didn't even realize the extent of her sleep issues until she got married. She thought it was normal to take a long time to fall asleep, toss and turn throughout the night, resort to sleep medication, and wake up tired. It wasn't until she began sleeping next to her husband that she observed that her habits were not shared by all. Her husband fell asleep easily, slept throughout the night without waking up, and woke up in the morning feeling well rested and energetic. It became abundantly clear that she needed to make some adjustments. Leslie had also battled depression and anxiety for years and was taking medication for both conditions. She committed to focusing on improving her sleep and put into action many of the steps discussed in this chapter. After several months of diligent attention, Leslie began to wean herself off the sleep medication. She started to fall asleep quickly after getting into bed and even slept through the night. She woke up rested and had energy that sustained her throughout the day. She felt better than she had for years. When Leslie tells her story, she admits that the adjustments she made were not easy. They took discipline and consistency, but the results were completely worthwhile. In addition to being far more productive, Leslie felt less depressed and less anxious.

ADVERSE EFFECTS OF SLEEP DEPRIVATION

Sleep deprivation affects cognitive function. Lack of sleep contributes to learning and problem-solving issues and can decrease both concentration and memory. When people don't get sufficient sleep, their neurons slow down.[77] When one has optimal sleep habits, there is a burst of electrical activity that brain cells use to communicate. When one is sleep deprived, this electrical activity becomes slower and weaker, which then leads to delayed behavioral responses and cognitive lapses. These cognitive lapses are serious enough to affect not only perception but reaction and memory. One's immune system is adversely affected by sleep deprivation. The likelihood of getting sick increases, and the recovery and healing time from getting sick take longer. Natural killer cells are thought to be lowered by as much as 79 percent after sleep deprivation. A study about the immune system during sleep confirms the association between the immune system and sleep, saying "sleep deprivation makes a living body susceptible to many infectious agents."[78] Appetite and metabolism are affected by inadequate sleep. Appetite increases, metabolism slows, and one has an increased risk for overeating, obesity, and type 2 diabetes. I have read that poor sleep can produce more insulin-related obesity than sugar consumption. Aging of the skin is accelerated and risks for emotional disorders, anxiety, and depression are all consequences of insufficient sleep. There are greater risks for high blood pressure, atherosclerosis, stroke, and heart failure as well as for several cancers.

It is noteworthy to point out that not only are there several organizations devoted exclusively to sleep research (American Sleep Association, National Center on Sleep Disorders Research, National Sleep Foundation), but at many of the top universities, there are entire departments, clinics, and laboratories focused exclusively on the subject and research of sleep. An interesting study concluded that sleeping less than seven hours a night correlated with a decrease in both physical and cognitive performance.[79] People lack the self-awareness to identify the negative implications of insufficient sleep. What happens is that people develop a misplaced belief that they adapt to fewer hours of sleep, when in fact, they do not realize the actual implications. For years, people have harbored misplaced pride about sleeping only a few hours each night. While there is a genetic predisposition to efficiency and high performance with only a few hours of sleep, this only applies to approximately 5 percent of the population.[80] There is about the same small percentage of the population who require a great deal of sleep to function effectively (greater than nine hours), but the majority of people require seven to nine hours of sleep.

Matthew Walker, the director of the Center for Human Sleep Science at the University of California, Berkeley, and the author of the bestselling book *Why We Sleep*, points out that "human beings are the only species that deliberately deprive themselves of sleep for no apparent gain."

CIRCADIAN RHYTHMS

One of our biological processes which have the greatest impact on our sleep is called the circadian rhythm. This process regulates all aspects of our health, including our sleep/wake cycle, our feeding cycles, our heart rate, our blood pressure, our hormone secretion, and our neurological function. These rhythms follow a twenty-four-hour cycle and when disrupted can result in a host of problems.

Further illustration of the importance of this concept is that in 2017, three Americans, Jeffrey C. Hall, Michael Rosbash, and Michael W. Young won the Nobel Prize "for their discoveries of molecular mechanisms controlling the circadian rhythm." They found the gene that led to a deeper understanding of circadian rhythms. This gene is called the "period" gene (mPER3), and a protein (PER) encoded by the gene increases at night and decreases during the day. Just like one's chronotype which is discussed later in this chapter, one's circadian rhythms cannot be changed since they are genetically determined. Both of these, however, can be modified.[81,82]

SUPRACHIASMATIC NUCLEUS (SCN)

Every cell in our body has its own circadian clock. These cells respond to changes in light and are programmed to turn our genes on and off at different times during the day and night. As Satchin Panda states in his book, *The Circadian Code,* "Circadian rhythms optimize biological functions. Every function in the body has a specific time because the body cannot accomplish all it needs to do at once." Panda goes on to explain that "the circadian clock is the body's internal timing system, which interacts with the timing of light and the food to produce our daily rhythms." The master clock which is in the hypothalamus portion of the brain is called the suprachiasmatic nucleus (SCN), and it controls most physiological responses, such as sleep/wake cycles, body temperature, and hormone regulation. Additionally, the job of the SCN is to guide and control the circadian clocks throughout the rest of our body, the peripheral clocks. The SCN works by detecting light entering through one's eyes. In the morning when we are exposed to sunlight, our eyes communicate with our bodies to wake up. At night after the sun sets, the darkness sends signals through our eyes to our body to get ready to sleep. When light enters the eyes, it hits the pineal gland which in turn controls the release of melatonin. I will go into the emerging field of "junk light" in another chapter and point out how it is contributing to circadian-rhythm dysfunction. The wrong spectrum of light at night interferes with the pineal gland's production of melatonin and can disrupt your sleep. Before the invention of the light bulb, people went to sleep and woke up according to the sun, moon, and natural light-and-dark cycles. As a result of so much artificial light dominating our lives, we no longer have a clear distinction between day and night.

We all go to sleep too late and wake up too early from time to time, and that is not cause for extreme worry. It is when poor sleep habits become consistent that cortisol levels increase, inflammation increases, and a litany of chronic diseases occur. As we approach middle age, our ability to endogenously produce melatonin begins to decline. Blood work on elderly people has shown that melatonin is nearly completely absent. It is frequently recommended to supplement with exogenous melatonin to reset one's dysfunctional circadian rhythms. Having said this, only do so under the guidance of a skilled practitioner. Never forget that we are all biochemically and genetically different. What works for one may not work at all for another. Despite all of the clinical studies concluding the many benefits of taking melatonin, I am unable to take this supplement. If I take even 0.5 mg, I feel like I have been heavily sedated, and I wake with a hangover. There is something odd with my individual biochemistry or genetics that makes this widely lauded supplement off limits for me.

Ideally, you want your external environment to match your internal biological clock. Examples of where this is not happening are shift work and jet lag. When we travel across different time zones our body clock gets disrupted. Both hormone secretion and body temperature change according to the body clock. When we sleep, our core body temperature decreases with the lowest degree occurring about two to three hours before waking. When we are flying across time zones, our bodies are controlling our body temperature according to the day-and-night cycle of our last location. The grogginess associated with jet lag is due to the daylight of your new location communicating with your brain that it should be awake, but your core temperature is decreased according to your previous location. The two conflicting messages result in a disoriented feeling.

Society is based on the routine of early rising. Most offices and other businesses start the day early in the morning, and school starts as early as 7:00 a.m. for some. As the old proverb goes, "the early bird catches the worm," which is an indication of the theory that early risers have a higher chance of success. Conventional wisdom has been that one can and must train themselves to get up early to achieve success. This was always a particular area of annoyance for me because when I was growing up, I was not an "early bird." I had a difficult time falling asleep at night and then an even more difficult time waking up in the morning. At one point in my schooling career, the headmaster of my school questioned why I was continually late to school, and he menacingly threatened to call me in the morning to wake me up. He did not expect me to respond by telling him that it would be quite helpful if he could call me in the morning to wake me up. He was only threatening me and, much to my disappointment, didn't call me to wake me up in the morning. He only chastised me regularly when I showed up to school after the morning bell.

CHRONOBIOLOGY

Michael Breus, PhD, is a clinical psychologist and a diplomate of the American Board of Sleep Medicine and has written a terrific book called *The Power of When.* Dr. Breus discovered that every person's biological clock is different. This should not really come as a surprise as we have learned that everyone is physiologically,

There is a relatively new area of science called "chronobiology." It focuses on the adaptation of humans to the solar and lunar cycles and is closely related to the field of circadian rhythms.

biochemically, and genetically different. Dr. Breus describes four basic chronotypes that describe most people. Depending on your specific chronotype, which is based on your own unique physiology, Dr. Breus believes that there are certain times of the day and night when you will be more effective in the pursuit of many different tasks. These include fitness, various health pursuits, sleep, work, eating, drinking, exercising creativity, pursuing money, and even having fun. It is believed that there is a perfect time to do everything, and when one identifies their chronotype, they can adjust their schedule and will operate at their maximum ability. If you think about it, it makes sense that you will be more productive and more effective if you can time your sleeping, eating, and other daily functions to be in alignment with your own natural circadian rhythms. This is exemplified by studies that conclude that there is a connection between the time one takes their medication and the corresponding influence on the DNA repair of their damaged cells. There is also a connection between when one eats and exercises and how timing of both of those activities can facilitate weight loss and improve fitness. Even the time of day when one commits to solving creative and analytical problems can result in greater success if aligned with one's chronobiology.

The four most common chronotypes identified by Dr. Breus are dolphins, lions, bears, and wolves.

DOLPHINS

Dolphins represent approximately 10 percent of the population. This type sleeps lightly and is prone to insomnia. Dolphins tend to be ruminators, type A personalities, and prone to anxiety. They are also described as having tendencies toward high intelligence and perfectionism.

LIONS

Lions represent approximately 15–20 percent of the population. This type is known for being early risers. Since lions wake up so early and are raring to go, they tend to tire in the late afternoon and have no trouble falling asleep easily and on the early side. Their most marked characteristics include being analytical and organized. While many lions are overachievers, they tend to avoid big risks.

BEARS

Bears represent approximately 50 percent of the population. This group does not have too many sleep issues, and they are most efficient from the middle of the morning into the early afternoon. Their sleep cycle is like that of the sun and they like a solid eight hours of sleep. They are not the ones who jump out of bed with a lot of energy, but rather they take some time to become alert after waking. They have steady energy and productivity and are balanced overall. They are described as being type B personalities, social, and risk averse.

WOLVES

Wolves represent approximately 15–20 percent of the population. This type is nocturnal, has difficulty waking up early, and performs best during the later hours of the day and night. Their defining characteristics include being fearless, impulsive, and insightful. Wolves are the risk-takers of the chronotype bunch and are known to be emotional and the iconoclasts of the world.

I definitely fell into the category of "wolves" for most of my life. Unfortunately, as I got older, my sleep habits, and perhaps even my chronotype, evolved. I don't think there is a chronotype that describes me currently. I must ponder deeply about the animal who represents my narrow window of productivity. This window of peak efficiency seems to be from about 10:00 a.m. to 11:30 a.m.!

As I learned about the defining characteristics of these different chronotypes, I thought about what it would be like to be each type. While each chronotype has some very impressive characteristics, each one also has some serious drawbacks. I imagine it's like most things in life in that there is good and bad about everything. While it may seem admirable to wake up at the crack of dawn if you have great difficulty waking up early, there are some negative aspects of the waking-early chronotype that seem less admirable. Rather than wish you could be a different type than what you genetically are, it is best to adjust your schedule to accommodate your natural peak times. If you are not inclined to read Dr. Breus's book, I highly recommend taking his online quiz to determine your chronotype. You can find it at www.thepowerofwhenquiz.com.

THE FIVE STAGES OF SLEEP

A chapter about sleep and how to optimize it would not be complete without a description of the five stages of sleep. Sleep is a complex biological process during which critical restoration occurs. During a good night's sleep, one experiences muscle repair, endocrine system optimization, memory consolidation, and brain detoxification.

Stage 1: The first stage of sleep is known as the transition phase. This is when you are at the beginning of your night's rest, and it typically lasts for only about five to ten minutes. During this stage of light sleep, you have rolling eye movements and your muscles begin to relax. Waking up during this stage is quite easy.

Stage 2: This stage represents about 50 percent of your night's rest and is still considered to be light sleep. During this stage, your eye movements stop, your muscles relax further, and your body temperature begins to decline. Your brain activity, heart rate, and breathing all slow down.

Stage 3: This stage is the beginning of deep sleep and is referred to as slow-wave sleep. It is NREM sleep or non-rapid eye movement sleep. One's brain waves are "delta waves" with occasional bursts of beta waves during this stage. In both this stage and the next one, hormones are secreted and blood flow to muscles is increased for repair. This is a hard stage of sleep to wake up from. As people get older, they spend less time in slow-wave deep sleep and more time in stage two light sleep.

Stage 4: During this stage, one experiences the deepest sleep. This is when the body performs most of its repair and regeneration. There are only delta waves during this period, and one's blood pressure drops and breathing slows further. While this typically lasts for just thirty minutes, it is optimal for it to represent 13–23 percent of your overall night's sleep. It is during this stage that the glymphatic system clears away metabolic waste accumulated throughout the day and performs the important function of detoxification.[83]

Stage 5: This is the only phase of sleep where the brain is highly active. This is active sleep. While one's limbs and muscles are still temporarily paralyzed, blood flow, breathing, and brain activity increase during this phase. It represents approximately 20–25 percent of your night's sleep, and it is when REM or rapid eye movement takes place. This stage usually begins about ninety minutes after you first fall asleep and is marked by several episodes. The early episodes last about ten minutes and the later episodes can last close to an hour. At the end of this stage, your body temperature begins to rise and you start to wake up.

SLEEP APNEA

While there are many factors contributing to inadequate sleep, sleep apnea and obstructive sleep apnea (OSA) really should be identified and remedied. Stress, medication, environment, and overall subpar lifestyle need to be remedied, but sleep apnea and OSA are factors that often continue undiagnosed and untreated. Sleep apnea results when your brain doesn't send the right signals to control your breathing. Obstructive sleep apnea is a result of upper airway obstruction. During both, breathing stops and starts throughout the night. Snoring is an indication that one's airways are collapsing. These disorders interfere with your restorative sleep, and the consequences of not treating them can be serious.

It should now be clear that nearly every system in the body, the immune system, the vascular system, and the endocrine system, as well as our microbiome and the repair of our damaged cells and tissues, are all adversely impacted by inadequate sleep.

When one prioritizes and takes steps to optimize their sleep, the result will be well worth the effort. Some of the steps you can take are as follows:

WAYS TO OPTIMIZE YOUR SLEEP ROUTINE

Consistent sleep and wake times are important to reset your circadian rhythms. When one goes to sleep at night, ideally it should be around ten to ten-thirty at night (unless you're a wolf chronotype!). The room in which you sleep should be as dark as you can handle and should be on the cool side of the thermostat. If you share your room with someone who has a different temperature tolerance than you, you can invest in a Chilipad, which is a device that circulates water and keeps you cool while not interrupting your sleep mate's temperature tolerance. It is important to research the best mattress for your preference. Above all, it should be nontoxic and not contain dangerous chemicals, which dominate the mattress industry. A couple of hours prior to sleeping, you should reduce or eliminate your exposure to electronic devices. The blue light emitted from these devices interferes with the production of your endogenous melatonin and growth hormone and can disrupt your sleep. There are glasses called "blue blocker" glasses which can help with the blocking of blue light. Be careful about relying on sleep medications because they can lead to dependence and have many negative side effects. It is best to avoid eating too close to sleep time as the process of digestion will interfere with your sleep. Avoid excessive alcohol because, while alcohol may assist in falling asleep, it interferes with the restorative aspects of sleep. A pink- or white-noise machine, or app on your phone, can help with falling asleep. Regular physical activity is of utmost importance not just for quality sleep but for many other reasons. It is also important for some to avoid caffeine later in the day. One usually knows what their individual caffeine tolerance is and should act accordingly. There are genes associated with the metabolization of caffeine and one could either be a fast or slow metabolizer. It is also believed that one should sleep at a slight incline because it facilitates lymphatic drainage if the head is propped up slightly. The degree of incline is small, about 5 percent.

In the morning, it is ideal to get morning light exposure within the first thirty to ninety minutes of waking. If you live in a location where this is not possible, there are several light boxes available for purchase that can serve as a substitute. This early light exposure will help with the balancing of your cortisol levels and reset your circadian rhythms, making it easier to fall asleep at night.

One method that I use to track my sleep performance is using a technological device called the Ōura Ring. I believe that one will achieve greater success in their quest for optimal health when they can track metrics. Using sensors embedded in the ring, the Ōura Ring can objectively measure your sleep metrics, activity level, heart rate variability, resting heart rate, and temperature. The sleep measurement function highlights your total sleep; your sleep efficiency defined as sleep quality; your restfulness, which is how restless you are throughout the night and how frequently you wake during the night; and the percentage of your REM sleep, deep sleep, and light sleep. It also provides a sleep latency score which tells you how long it took to fall asleep. Using a device like this provides motivation to focus and prioritize your sleep habits.

The costs of sleep deprivation are great, and the benefits of optimizing your sleep are valuable.

ACTION STEPS

➤ Set consistent going-to-sleep and waking-up times and adhere to them.

➤ Make your bedroom as dark as possible. Block out as much incoming light as you can. Cover up little lights emanating from TVs and other devices.

➤ Make your bedroom temperature sixty-two to sixty-eight degrees.

➤ Invest in a Chilipad or other similar device if your sleeping partner can't tolerate sleeping in a room with a cool temperature.

➤ Incorporate breathwork before going to sleep if you have difficulty falling asleep. (See chapter 9.)

➤ Optimize blue- and red-light exposure. (See chapter 12.)

➤ Reduce nighttime exposure to devices.

➤ Invest in a nontoxic mattress and pillow.

➤ Briefly expose your eyes to sunlight within the first thirty to ninety minutes of waking. If you live in the Northern latitude, invest in a light box.

CHAPTER 7

NUTRITION:
You Are What You Eat

IT IS AN UNDERSTATEMENT TO say that there is a lack of consensus in nutritional science. Some of this confusion is perpetuated by the food industry, the scientists, and the media. The confusion regarding nutritional science has many contributing factors. It is in part due to the profit motive of the food industry which places their financial motives over the health of their consumers. There is also the factor of policy influences. Our federal government subsidizes the growing of corn, soy, and other crops.[84] Yet another factor making it difficult to rely on this field is that it turns out that it is exceedingly difficult to conduct accurate clinical studies on nutrition. Everyone has different genetic and physiological responses to food, and that is not considered. People have to self-report as participants of nutritional studies, and they tend to do so inaccurately. There is a great deal of cherry-picking of the data by whoever is sponsoring the study to achieve desired results.

> Food is one of the most important factors of your health and one of the most complicated areas of science.

THE KEY TO YOUR HEALTH SPAN

Despite the confusion as to what to eat, how much to eat, and when to eat, Hippocrates is thought to have stated, "Let food be thy medicine and let medicine be thy food." Today this is confirmed by the increasing belief that food is the ultimate pharmacology. It is literally the key to one's health span. Every single bit of food we choose to eat is either contributing to our health or hurting our health. The foods that one chooses to eat have the potential to change your gene expression, your hormonal balance, and your critical metabolic function. Food can switch on or switch off genes. As the science of epigenetics evolves further, it will have an enormous impact on the science of nutrition. Food can either promote health or it can lead to illness.

> The role of nutrition is to build up your own natural defense system, and many believe that if our population changed how they ate, many more lives would be saved than using a vaccine or pharmaceuticals.

A current-day physician and professor of pharmacology, Dr. Louis Ignarro, continues Hippocrates's concept by conducting his own research into the association between nutrition and disease. Dr. Ignarro is a Nobel laureate in medicine and has written a compelling book called *Health Is Wealth*. The book is a result of Dr. Ignarro being swayed away from his conventional medical education focused on pharmaceuticals for treating disease. He looked at thousands of scientific studies that illustrated that food can, indeed, function as medicine. His book "examine[s] nutrient interactions within the body's biochemical pathways and physiological functions" and supports "the idea that our current disease-care system must be replaced [...]."

MACRONUTRIENTS VS. MICRONUTRIENTS

Macronutrients include carbohydrates, protein, and fat. Each has its own function in the body. Carbohydrates provide us with energy. Protein contributes to immune and gut function, muscle building, and tissue repair. Fat is the preferred source of energy, and it also assists in cell membrane function and regulates hormone production. Micronutrients are vitamins and minerals that are required for the efficient metabolic function of our body. I describe them in greater detail in chapter 15.

SOIL DEPLETION

While there are many issues plaguing the area of nutrition, a critical one is the decline of nutritional value in the food being produced today. Even if one chooses to eat a healthy diet filled with fruits, vegetables, and other whole foods, there is the problem of soil depletion. Decades ago, people could obtain all the vitamins, minerals, and nutrients that they needed from the food they ate. This is no longer possible as industrial agriculture has contributed to the change of the nutritional value of our food supply.

Along with the glyphosate and other pesticides sprayed on the crops, the soil no longer contains important minerals and nutrients. The result of this is the production of food lacking in the all-important nutrient density. There is one study that showed that you would have to eat as many as eight oranges today to get the same vitamin A content as

The intent of industrial agriculture was originally to produce more crops to feed more people. The problem with that is the higher yield cultivation of crops has resulted in more crops with far less nutritional value.

a single orange yielded years ago. Another study confirmed that a tomato grown by conventional farming today has nearly no lycopene left in it. Dr. Phil Warman, an agronomist and professor of agricultural sciences at Nova Scotia Agricultural College, states that "crops are bred to produce higher yields, to be resistant to disease and to produce more visually attractive fruits and vegetables, but little or no emphasis is placed on their vitamin and mineral content."

In 1987, Brazil hosted a global conference on the environment and concluded that nearly 90 percent of the topsoil had been depleted. This was thirty-three years ago, and it's worse today, with a clear connection between pesticides, fungicides, and herbicides contributing to accelerated aging and the amount of disease.

A triple board-certified doctor named Zach Bush has said that we have only sixty crop yields left in this country before the soil becomes devoid of all minerals and nutrients. He studies the role of soil and water in human health and is genuinely concerned about today's agricultural practices and their destruction of our soils, water systems, oceans, and human health. In addition to the dire effect on nutrients in food, this will affect the earth's ability to filter water, absorb carbon, and feed the world's population.

GLYPHOSATE

The soil issue requires a discussion of glyphosate and GMO crops. This is a controversial area, with many insisting that GMO crops are safe. In a nutshell, GMO crops are genetically modified organisms where a foreign gene has been inserted into plants so they will become more resistant to threats, like weed killers. The goal was to spray a weed killer such as Roundup (glyphosate) around the crops to kill the weeds but to leave the crops unharmed by the weed "killer." The unintended consequences of this approach were to taint not only the soil but also the crops because there is no way that the spraying, even with the best of intentions, didn't land on the crops. You cannot get rid of glyphosate. You can't wash it off, and it's on non-GMO crops now also. Most pigs, cows, and chickens eat glyphosate-sprayed corn and grain, so if you eat these animals, you are ingesting glyphosate as well.[85,86,87,88] Some residue of the spraying remains on GMO crops which adversely affects your gut microbiome. The crops which are the worst offenders are the non-GMO wheat and oats which are sprayed with Roundup just before harvest to dry them (a process called desiccation). The products that are made from these crops have the highest levels of this toxin.

Just recently, the first case against Monsanto for Roundup causing a man's cancer resulted in a win. There have been many more cases filed since that one, and the company Monsanto was purchased by Bayer. The company, formerly known as Monsanto, now operates under the name of Bayer to gain distance from the association of cancer-causing Roundup and Monsanto. The connection between pesticides, weed killers, chemical fertilizers made from petroleum, and disease is clear. This litigation revealed that the formulations of the herbicide caused the most toxicity and carcinogenicity and the problems did not arise from glyphosate alone.

METABOLIC DYSFUNCTION

As I write this, we are amid the COVID-19 pandemic. Another equally, if not more serious epidemic is that of metabolic dysfunction. It is prevalent among the US population and is spreading worldwide. For some reason, this extremely dangerous epidemic gets insufficient attention.

I don't believe that we will have a true picture of the COVID virus until after it no longer presents a global health issue, I do believe that the metabolic health of those who died and those who had serious responses to the virus will play a large part. We evolved during

Dr. Dariush Mozaffarian, dean of the Friedman School of Nutrition Science and Policy at Tufts University, has stated that "fewer than one American adult in five is metabolically healthy" and that "poor diet is now the leading cause of poor health in the U.S., causing more than half a million deaths per year."

a period of food scarcity accompanied by the need to move about frequently. Today, it is the opposite. There is an abundance of food, though not well distributed to those who are food insecure, and an increase in a sedentary lifestyle. These factors are responsible for the growing epidemic of metabolic syndrome defined by type 2 diabetes, cardiovascular disease, obesity, and other diseases of inflammation. These chronic diseases are killing us in large numbers, and they barely existed years ago. I would be remiss in failing to acknowledge the numerous improvements in the quality of life today, but they are offset by the fact that life expectancy is declining as these metabolic diseases increase. This crisis is described as a major health hazard that is imposing unsustainable costs to health care and loss of potential economic activity. The causes of metabolic syndrome are a result of the increase of unhealthy food consumption while physical activity is decreasing.[89]

WE EAT TOO MUCH, TOO OFTEN

The numbers are staggering, and I have noted them throughout this book. While it may be irritating to be repetitive, certain dire situations bear repeating. Today, 70.7 percent of Americans are overweight with 38 percent of those being obese. This is largely due in part to the Standard American Diet, known as SAD, but also due to other factors, such as how frequently one eats and even when one eats. We are a nation that loves to snack. Some time ago, we were advised to eat three meals and two snacks a day. Perhaps, if you suffer from hypoglycemia or need to maintain a steady glucose balance for a particular reason, more frequent small meals may be in order, but for most of us, we are eating too much, too often. Every time you eat, you release insulin because your metabolism burns glucose before burning fat. Your digestive system doesn't get sufficient time to rest and repair if there aren't enough hours between eating. When you are hungry, your body's repair mechanisms are triggered. Not only does the frequency of eating affect you adversely, but the timing of eating can as well. There was a study conducted by the American Heart Association which concluded that the timing of your food intake may affect your risk profile for cardiovascular and metabolic diseases. It was found that you should get most of your calories earlier in the day and have a light dinner. Eating most of your calories after six in the evening increases your risk for disease.[90] This is explained by the concept of circadian clocks and your response to food intake. Periods of time without eating, preferably at night, can reset your clock gene rhythms. As mentioned before, Professor Satchidananda Panda of the Salk Institute in California wrote a book called *The Circadian Code* where he goes into detail about the mechanisms of meal timing. He believes that eating should be restricted to an eight-to-ten-hour window.

THE LESS YOU EAT, THE LONGER YOU LIVE

Before we begin the extremely broad topic of what to eat, it's important to cover the optimal amount of food to eat. There are studies supporting that caloric restriction is an effective way to delay aging and increase longevity.[91,92] This has been known for decades and is associated with a clear reduction in the risk of cardiovascular disease and cancer. Reducing one's caloric intake puts mild stress, or hormetic stress, on the body which results in a positive adaptation of cellular repair. The amount that one eats has a direct effect on mTOR. mTOR stands for mammalian target of rapamycin and is a protein that regulates cell growth and metabolism. mTOR increases after eating and decreases during fasting.[93] mTOR is a regulator of aging. If you are concerned about aging, and really, who isn't, you want to inhibit excessive mTOR. The key is to avoid overdoing it and to avoid starving oneself. One should attempt this by reducing their normal caloric intake and, at the same time, taking care to avoid a drastic reduction of essential nutrients. This method should only be done occasionally to avoid adverse effects.

THE DOWNFALL OF DIETS

There is an endless debate in nutrition over the appropriate ratio of macronutrients. Macronutrients are carbohydrates, fats, and proteins, and are the basis of the most structured diets. There are low-carb, high-fat, high-protein diets; high-carb, low-protein, and low-fat diets; and every other possible combination. There is the ketogenic diet, the paleo diet, the carnivore diet, the vegetarian diet, the vegan diet, what Dr. Mark Hyman calls the "pegan diet," and countless more. Personally, I do not believe in the long-term efficacy of diets. Most of them are fads based on faulty science and dogma, and while they may result in initial weight loss, chances are good that the weight loss is just temporary and one will either plateau or worse, gain the weight back. This is in part due to compliance but more due to our individual genetic and physiological differences. What works great for your friend may not work at all for you. You likely are unaware of your genetic markers and if you carry certain genetic variations, for example, the ketogenic diet may be wholly inappropriate for you. Certain genes are not compatible with high levels of fat and even though you may lose weight and even feel good, chances are that you are unaware of your internal responses.

YOU WANT A FLEXIBLE METABOLISM

Diet success depends on the purpose of the diet. Is the purpose for weight loss or for improving one's general health and reducing disease risk? If the goal is weight loss, there are two main factors. One is the maintenance of steady blood sugar and the avoidance of glucose spikes. This requires some due diligence on the part of the individual because we all respond differently to food. A continuous glucose monitor is a tremendous tool to gain insight into this factor. This is the best way I know of to monitor your individual response to each thing that you eat. After collecting this critical information, you can adjust your diet accordingly. The second main factor in weight loss is feeling satisfied, or satiety. This is where caloric restriction presents problems. It is difficult to be satisfied when you aren't eating very much! If you restrict your calories too much and neglect eating nutrient-dense food, you can negatively affect your metabolism, slow it down, and sabotage your efforts. So, while weight loss is known to occur when you consume less energy than you expend, it is a delicate balance. Metabolism is tricky. You don't want a slow metabolism, and you don't want a fast metabolism either. Ideally, you want a flexible metabolism. The metabolism is an adaptive and reactive system. If you restrict your caloric intake too much or for too long of a time, your metabolism will compensate by reduced function and will become more rigid and less flexible.

If your dietary goal is less about weight loss and more about optimizing your overall health, you want to emphasize whole, not processed foods, healthy fats, restrict glucose, and include a diverse selection of foods. A healthy diet can optimize your immune system, which is an important goal. There is so much conflicting information about the appropriate amount of protein that one must attempt to discern what's best for their own physiology. On the one hand, several articles are proclaiming that the consumption of too much protein accelerates aging and there are just as many articles stating that inadequate amounts of protein can cause sarcopenia, or muscle loss, and result in harm for elderly people.[94]

ELIMINATION DIETS

One effective way to do your own due diligence and determine your responses to food, including food sensitivities and intolerances is the elimination diet. Apparently, somewhere between 2–20 percent of the population suffers from food intolerances. Often, the symptoms which include internal inflammation are difficult to identify and are even more difficult to associate with a particular food or cause. Some symptoms of food intolerances include joint and muscle pain, weight gain, brain fog, fatigue, skin issues/rashes, digestive issues, hair loss, depression, anxiety, and sinus issues. You begin by eliminating the foods which are known to be most problematic such as gluten, dairy, sugar, nuts, seafood, and others that you may suspect as problem causing. The elimination phase should last for about two to three weeks. Once the elimination phase ends, you want to introduce each food that has been eliminated one by one. After approximately four to five days, reintroduce another food and track your symptoms.

MISLEADING FOOD LABELING

Delving into the voluminous bad news surrounding nutrition, it's important to cover food labeling. There is no shortage of trickiness in food labeling. The term "organic" is a term regulated by the USDA, but it does not mean that a food item with this designation is wholly without pesticides. For one thing, this certification allows for certain less harmful pesticides to be used. It is exceedingly difficult to prevent the wind from carrying pesticides from a nonorganic farm to a nearby "organic" farm. Rain runoff can also carry soil tainted with pesticides to nearby farms and into the water supply. Another issue with foods labeled as organic is that both conventional manure and sludge from wastewater contain cadmium. Both the tainted manure and the tainted water are used to water the allegedly "organic" crops. In California, it's considered legal to use fracking fluids for growing food. Much of the food labeled as organic in the grocery stores is from China and can be ladened with heavy metals along with other pesticides. Ideally, the label "biodynamic certification" should be on the foods you consume. Terms like "farm raised," "responsibly made," "sustainable," "mom approved," and "all natural" are not regulated and can end up meaning nothing at all. These are called "healthwashing" or "greenwashing" and should not be relied upon. Examples of the misleading nature of food labeling are seen in the poultry and livestock industry. The term "free range" only means that, at some point, the animal was allowed to go outside. It fails to address the fact that the animal could be given antibiotics, hormones, fed GMO grain, and kept in a crowded area for most of their lives. In the US, chickens cannot be given hormones, but cows can be given hormones. Chickens in the US can be labeled "antibiotic free" as long as the residue tests under the certain "parts per billion" threshold the government has established. So a chicken labeled antibiotic-free could have been given antibiotics from birth to death as long as it was under a threshold amount. The term "cage free" simply means that the birds are raised outside of a cage, but they could be in horribly overcrowded spaces in factory farms. The most reliable label is "pasture raised from local farmers." Then, you just need to concern yourself with the existence of arsenic found in chickens. The FDA admitted in 2015 that 70 percent of chickens sold for human consumption in the US contain arsenic, which is carcinogenic, poisonous, and a hormone disruptor. The source of this arsenic is the grain that is fed to the chickens, hence the expression, "You are what the animal you eat ate." Arsenic has also been found in rice, mushrooms, and wine.

Still under the category of deceptive labeling are the methods used to conceal the amount of sugar in a product. It is almost without controversy that sugar is toxic, and we do not need to consume

Other names for sugar:

Barley malt, Barbados sugar, Evaporated Cane Juice, Brown sugar, Buttered syrup, Cane juice, Cane sugar, Caramel, Corn syrup[, Corn syrup solids, Confectioner's sugar, Carob syrup, Beet sugar, Castor sugar, Date sugar, Dehydrated cane juice, Demerara sugar, Dextran, Dextrose, Diastatic malt, Diastase, Ethyl maltol, Sorghum syrup, Fructose, Fruit juice, Syrup, Lactose, Maltose, High Fructose corn syrup(HFCS), Glucose, Glucose solids, Golden sugar, Golden syrup, Galactose, Honey, Icing sugar, Invert sugar, Starch, Malt, Maltodextrin, Fruit juice concentrate, Malt syrup, Mannitol, Maple syrup, Molasses, Muscovado, Panocha, Powdered sugar, Raw sugar, Refiner's sugar, Table sugar, Rice syrup, Sorbitol, Free flowing brown sugars, Sucrose, Granulated sugar, Treacle, Turbinado sugar, Yellow sugar, Agave nectar, Cane crystals, Corn sweetener, Crystalline fructose, Maltotroise.[95]

it. The food manufacturers know this, too, and go to great lengths to hoodwink us into thinking that there is less sugar in products than we think. Ingredients are listed with the highest amount of any ingredient at the top and then continue in descending order. There are many kinds of sweeteners including high-fructose corn syrup, regular corn syrup, honey, maple syrup, agave, brown rice syrup, fructose, dextrose, maltose, sucrose, trehalose, isoglucose, isomaltose, and others. One can easily buy a product without the words "cane sugar" on the ingredient list thinking it isn't high in sugar content. In fact, all of the other types of sweeteners cause similar glucose reactions in your body. If you recall how the tobacco industry deceived the population for years, the deception of the sugar industry is quite similar. It is truly remarkable how the greed of the food industry threatens our health.

THE FOOD LOBBY DOES NOT CARE ABOUT OUR HEALTH

The next area of deception in nutrition has to do with the food lobby and food scientists. The food lobby is rich and powerful and often uses its power in nefarious ways. Their first concern is the companies that they represent and the financial profits from the sale of food products. They appear to have little, if any, concern for the health of the consumer, which is usually at odds with the profit motive. One glaring example of this is the food lobby's success in convincing the FDA to allow the labeling of a food product "trans-fat free" if it contains less than 0.5 grams of trans fat per serving. Trans fats are the worst fats one can consume, and they are known to increase inflammation and cardiovascular disease. Trans fats are a form of unsaturated fat that is made through the chemical process of the hydrogenation of oils. They are found in processed foods such as baked goods, snack foods, fried foods, nondairy coffee creamer, microwave popcorn, frozen pizza, shortening, margarine, and certain vegetable oils. The American Heart Association issued a recommendation that one should limit their intake of trans fat to less than 2 grams per day. Personally, I think one should avoid them altogether. The issue is that 0.5 grams add up, and people are not given transparent information when they think the product they're consuming is, in fact, trans-fat free as the label states. It makes you wonder, how else are we being deceived?

While I would like to believe that all food scientists, technologists, and chemists are not bad, many have been co-opted by the evils of the food industry. Instead of focusing on the nutritious value of food, many are hired to manipulate different food ingredients like sugar, salt, and fat to influence our chemistry of addiction. In his book called *Salt Sugar Fat*, Michael Moss, the Pulitzer Prize winner, illustrates how ingredients are engineered to encourage people to become addicted to unhealthy foods. The entire process, intending to create a dependency, seems quite sinister to me. This is a clear contributor to our US epidemic of obesity.

FOOD ADDITIVES

Food additives are another category of deception and harm. If the ingredients listed on a package are not familiar or you need to look them up to understand them, do not buy the food. If the ingredient has a color or a number next to it, it is a chemical and most probably should not be ingested. If it is hard to pronounce and has multiple syllables, it's probably a chemical and shouldn't be ingested. If it is all capital letters, like BHA, it's a chemical formulation. If the label on the package says that the product has been enriched, that means that the food has been stripped of its naturally occurring nutrients and replaced by chemical formulations. There is a terrific book called *Feeding You Lies* by Vani Hari, a food activist. Her book reveals how nutritional research is manipulated, the dangers of food additives, and misleading information disseminated by the food industry. Hari has been successful in persuading several big food companies like Kraft, Chick-fil-A, Subway, General Mills, and Starbucks to remove harmful additives and to become more transparent about their ingredients. Artificial colors can disrupt the immune system, are banned in some countries, and can be contaminated with carcinogens. Despite this information, artificial colors remain in a lot of foods. Most flour contains a chemical additive called bromine. This additive has a long list of health issues including being potentially carcinogenic, causing DNA damage, causing skin irritations, thyroid problems, and mental problems. These issues occur frequently enough so that there is a disorder called bromism. King Arthur is a brand of flour that is not bromated. Similarly, it's a good idea to find a baking powder that doesn't contain aluminum. Rumford is one brand that is aluminum free.

THE SAFEST FISH TO EAT

When buying fish to eat, your best bet is to buy wild-caught fish. Farmed fish is fed corn and given antibiotics among other things you would be better off avoiding. If you must eat farmed fish, salmon from Canada, especially from British Columbia, have fewer toxins than fish farmed in the US. The safest farmed fish are believed to come from Chile. There is a USDA database online which lists the nutrients in farmed and wild fish. The highest mercury content is found in the biggest fish, such as shark, swordfish, king mackerel, tuna, orange roughy, marlin, Chilean sea bass, lobster, halibut, and snapper. Smaller fish like anchovies, sardines, and wild-caught Alaskan salmon are among the fish with the least amount of methylmercury.

The EPA (Environmental Protection Agency) has local advisories for the mercury content of fish in different areas. It is advised to look for the logo MSC, which signifies Marine Stewardship Council, when buying wild fish. When buying farmed fish, look for the label BAP, which signifies global aquaculture practices were used. Alaska has a process whereby the chain of custody begins with the catching of the fish and continues all the way to the arrival at the store. Apparently, this chain of custody is strictly supervised. Costco, Trader Joe's, Walmart, and Whole Foods are stores that are known to be stringent with their fish standards. Having said all of this, it bears mentioning that the seafood industry is rife with fraud. A nonprofit marine conservation group called Oceana conducted a study on fraud in the seafood industry and found that in New York City, fraud existed in 58 percent of retail stores and 39 percent of restaurants. The way that this presents is by fish sold as a premium species when, in fact, it is a different type of fish. This is not only economic fraud, but it can also have dangerous health implications. There is a fish called escolar which contains a natural wax ester and can give people digestive distress for days. In the book *Real Food Fake Food* by Larry Olmsted, the US Government Accountability Office is quoted as saying, "Most seafood buyers [...] assume that the seafood they buy is what the seller claims it is. However, this is not always the case. Sometimes seafood products are mislabeled for financial gain—an activity called seafood fraud. [...] [This] fraud can result in food safety problems."

SUGAR

The list of foods to avoid is long, and I will cover the most egregious ones. Sugar is known to be toxic. Gary Taubes, a journalist, has written several books about nutrition but none as inflammatory about the use of sugar in the US as his book called *The Case Against Sugar*. Sugar is believed to be a core driver of every major disease including diabetes, cancer, cardiovascular disease, autoimmune disease, and depression. Fructose is the worst kind of sugar as it turns into fat in your body faster than any other kind of sugar and increases your risk of insulin resistance. Agave nectar is bad also as it is 90 percent fructose.

PROCESSED OILS

As bad as sugar is, processed oil is much worse and is just becoming acknowledged for the havoc it wreaks on human health. For years, we thought cooking with and using vegetable seed oils was great for our health. Like so many other instances, we were sold the wrong bill of goods. The seed oils which should be banished from your home include canola, corn, cottonseed, soybean, sunflower, safflower, peanut, sesame, and rice bran oil. There are several issues with these highly industrialized oils. They are low cost, low quality, chemically unstable, highly processed, and increase inflammation and your risk of chronic disease. The method used to process these oils involves refining, bleaching, using a petroleum-based solvent called hexane, and then adding some more chemicals. When the oils are heated and then reheated, the molecules change and toxic byproducts are released. This causes free radicals to form followed by oxidative stress and DNA damage.[96] A major issue contributing to the harm of these oils is the imbalance of omega-6 to omega-3 fatty acids. These are called polyunsaturated fatty acids, or PUFAs. Omega-6 fatty acids are pro-inflammatory and, while we need some of them, we don't need as many as are in these oils. Omega-3 fatty acids are anti-inflammatory, and the ratio of the two is ideally one to one. These seed oils have caused the increase of this one-to-one ratio to about ten or twenty to one, favoring the pro-inflammatory omega-6s. Linoleic acid is the main chemical compound found in omega-6s in seed oils and has been associated with oxidative stress, increased inflammation, and coronary artery disease.[97] Many studies are emerging that suggest that the imbalance of omega-6 to omega-3 fatty acids is a contributor to Alzheimer's disease, dementia, cancer, cardiovascular disease, depression, gut issues, diabetes, obesity, and arthritis.[98] Some studies have revealed that soybean oil causes not only metabolic diseases like diabetes but also contributes to adverse changes in the brain. Evidently, soybean oil has been found by researchers to affect the hypothalamus and to cause the dysregulation of about a hundred genes.

BENEFICIAL OILS

The good news is that oils like olive oil, coconut oil, and avocado oil, if unprocessed and organic, can be quite beneficial to your overall health. Olive oil increases a component of HDL, the good cholesterol called apoA-IV. This component reduces blood clotting in arteries by preventing platelets from sticking together and lowers the risk of cardiovascular disease. Another valuable benefit of consuming olive oil is its reduction of inflammation and lowering the risk of osteoporosis. It is filled with antioxidants and polyphenols.

It is low in saturated fat and high in omega-3 fatty acids that reduce the risk of disease.

A little bit of bad news in the olive oil story is that fake olive oil is abundant on the market. Not only can the fake olive oil be unhealthy, but some of it also isn't even made from olives.[99] There are several ways to sell fake olive oil, but the main ways that can potentially harm your health are the dilution with less expensive, processed seed oils; the dilution with lower grades of olive oil which have been chemically refined; and adding old, rancid olive oil to new olive oil. One should buy olive oil from reputable companies or, if possible, directly from the farms producing the oil.

DAIRY PRODUCTS

People love dairy products and are often unaware of the problems associated with dairy consumption. Conventionally raised cows are given hormones to fatten them up and increase their milk production. Conventionally raised cows are fed GMO soy, GMO corn, and cottonseed, all of which are laced with pesticides, antibiotics, and sometimes even chicken manure. These practices expose people who consume dairy to things they should avoid. Contrary to popular belief, people can't easily digest the calcium from cow milk. Due to the process of homogenization of most milk, the proteins are denatured thereby making them difficult to digest. The pasteurization process of milk kills good bacteria and enzymes along with the harmful bacteria it is intended to kill. This also adversely impacts the digestion of milk and dairy products. After the age of five years old, we no longer produce the necessary enzymes for breaking down lactose and milk proteins. Whey protein from milk, which is in a lot of protein powders, contains a lot of estrogen. One can experience fatigue, bloating, and abdominal fat when using this kind of whey protein for prolonged amounts of time. Speaking of protein powders, one should be wary of the ingredients. Soy lecithin and maltodextrin are just two ingredients frequently found in commercial protein powders which are inflammatory and cause blood sugar spikes.

GLUTEN

Gluten is a hotbed of controversy when it comes to food issues. There is celiac disease which is a condition where the protein gluten causes an auto-immune response of the body attacking the small intestine. This disorder affects about 1 percent of the American population and can be confirmed with testing. Then there is non-celiac gluten sensitivity (NCGS), or just gluten sensitivity, where the body experiences digestive and nondigestive symptoms (headaches, joint pain, fatigue, brain fog, skin issues, and mood issues) after consuming food containing gluten. There is no actual test to confirm this disorder, and doctors disagree as to its existence.

Gluten Foods and Ingredients That Contain Gluten[100]

Wheat, Barley (malt), Rye, Oats, Triticale, Spelt, Durum (semolina), Einkorn, Emmer, Groat, Graham, Beer, Malted Beverages, Grain based spirits, Artificial colors, Artificial flavors, Baking powder, Bouillon cubes or stock cubes, candy may be dusted with wheat flour, some canned soups, Caramel color and flavoring, Cheese spreads and other processed cheese foods, Chocolate-may contain malt flavoring, Cold cuts, Wieners, ,Sausages-may contain gluten due to cereal fillers, Dextrin, Dip mixes, Dry roasted nuts and honey roasted nuts, Dry sauce mixes, Extenders and binders, French fries in restaurants, Gravies(thickening agent and liquid base), Honey hams-can be based with wheat starch in coating, Hydrogenated Starch Hydrolysate, Hydrolyzed plant protein, Hydrolyzed vegetable protein, Hydroxy propylated Starch, Instant Teas & Coffees (cereal products may be included in the formulation), MSG, Maltodextrin (wheat or corn based), Maltose, Mayonnaise-check thickener and grain based vinegar ingredients, Miso, Modified food starch, Mustard-mustard powder may contain gluten, Natural colors, Natural flavors, Non Dairy Creamer, Pregelatinized starch, Seasonings-check labels, Smoke flavors, Soy Sauce, Textured vegetable protein, Vegetable gum, Vegetable protein, Vitamin supplements-some have grain based ingredients, stamps and envelopes, toothpaste, lipstick, Hairspray & Shampoo, Detergents, Pet Food, Medications, Lotions, Play dough and Makeup

The only treatment for either disorder is to refrain from consuming anything with gluten as an ingredient. This is easier said than done because gluten is ubiquitous. It is in products that you would never suspect, often used as a filler. Gluten is even used as a binding agent in certain prescription and over-the-counter medications. The grains containing gluten are barley, einkorn, emmer, farro, Kamut, rye, spelt, triticale, and wheat. It is in several flours, alcohols, and even things like artificial colors, sauces, ground spices and seasonings, oats, soy sauce, and other things that would never be considered problematic.

The most common and frequently consumed food which contains gluten is wheat. The way that wheat is produced and processed today is quite different from fifty years ago. Most of the wheat today has been genetically modified to increase yield and to resist pests. The result of this alteration in wheat is adverse food reactivity. It is believed that the gluten symptoms are a result of gut permeability, which occurs because humans cannot completely digest gluten. Alessio Fasano, MD, a celiac researcher at Massachusetts General Hospital, has written a book called *Gluten*

Freedom. In this book, he explains that the smaller protein in gluten, called gliadin, causes the release of zonulin, a protein that regulates gut permeability and is associated with leaky gut. When one's
gut becomes leaky, bacteria, toxins, and undigested food are free
to enter directly into the bloodstream, causing inflammation. He
also explains that gluten causes antibodies to form which contribute to inflammation and can cause autoimmune disease. Gluten is
also thought to trigger neurochemical changes in the production of
neurotransmitters. Gluten is shown to be a neurotoxin that damages
nerve tissue.

FILLERS

Speaking of gut permeability, fillers in nut milks and other foods
include carrageenan and guar gum, both known to increase inflammation and digestive issues. Many food additives that are banned in
other countries are allowed in the US and have been shown to cause
digestive issues. Some of these are xanthan gum, cellulose gum, lecithin, polysorbate 80, and carboxymethylcellulose. Polysorbate 80,
along with propylene glycol are in "natural" flavors. There is nothing natural about either of those. Be very wary of "natural flavors."
MSG is another conundrum. The number of alternative names for
monosodium glutamate could be considered creative if it wasn't so
sneaky. MSG is a flavor enhancer linked to a litany of health issues. It
is frequently processed in a way where it is no longer 99 percent pure
and therefore is not required by the FDA to be listed as an ingredient. Be on the lookout for the following names indicating the presence of MSG: yeast extract, textured vegetable protein, hydrolyzed
vegetable protein (or anything hydrolyzed), glutamic acid, glutamate, monopotassium glutamate, calcium gluconate, magnesium
gluconate, natrium gluconate, calcium caseinate, sodium caseinate,
gelatin, textured protein, soy protein isolate, whey protein isolate,

vetsin, carrageenan, bouillon and broth, stock, any flavors or flavoring, maltodextrin, anything ultra-pasteurized, barley malt, pectin, protease, malt extract, soy sauce, seasonings.

MSG Names[101]

Acid hydrolyzed vegetable protein, Autolyzed Yeast, Hydrolyzed corn protein, HVP, hydrolyzed casein, hydrolyzed collagen, hydrolyzed collagen protein, hydrolyzed corn, hydrolyzed corn soy wheat gluten protein, hydrolyzed cornstarch, hydrolyzed gelatin, hydrolyzed milk protein, hydrolyzed oat flour, Hydrolyzed Plant Protein, hydrolyzed soy, hydrolyzed soybean protein, hydrolyzed torula and brewers yeast protein, hydrolyzed vegetable protein, hydrolyzed wheat, hydrolyzed whey protein, hydrolyzed yeast, MSG, partially hydrolyzed beef stock, partially hydrolyzed casein, partially hydrolyzed guar gum, partially hydrolyzed soybean, partially hydrolyzed whey protein, Plant Protein Extract, Textured Protein, Yeast Extract

Consuming soy and other soy products is safe to do if it's organic (edamame or tofu) or fermented (miso, tempeh, and tamari). It's prudent to avoid any soy product that has undergone ultra-processing. This includes fake meats and cheeses made from processed soy, soy additives, and soy protein isolate which is a powder from soybeans that is processed using the solvent hexane. Coffee is another item to consider. Conventional coffee is among the most chemically treated foods. It is made up of fertilizers, pesticides, herbicides, fungicides, and insecticides. Due to the way the coffee beans are stored, most are contaminated with mycotoxins or mold. It is worth buying organic, carefully sourced coffee.

FINALLY, GOOD NEWS!

And now, for some good news. As harmful to our health as certain foods can be, other foods can be healing and health promoting. Fruits, vegetables, and some herbs and spices contain polyphenols which are bioactive plant compounds. These are both antioxidants and anti-inflammatory. The darker the color of the fruit or vegetable, the higher content of polyphenolic molecules. Wild plants are stressed plants because they grow in imperfect conditions and must develop natural defense mechanisms. When you eat these plants, you increase your ability to mount your antioxidant defense. The polyphenols impart resilience to the plants and to those who eat the plants. They communicate with your genes to activate longevity and other beneficial pathways. Food truly is information.

EGGS

Eggs confuse me. I have read as many articles and studies vilifying the consumption of eggs as I have glorifying eggs. I suspect, like everything else, it comes down to one's individual response. For some, eggs may present an issue. In any event, they are known to be rich in the antioxidants lutein and zeaxanthin. They are nutrient dense and filled with vitamins B2, B12, D, choline, iron, and selenium. Many of the studies which declared that eating eggs raises your cholesterol were sponsored by the cereal board! This is just one more example of how we have been misled when it comes to nutrition. Cholesterol is the precursor of different steroid hormones like cortisol and testosterone. Not long ago, an article in the Harvard Medical School newsletter reflected that unlike years ago when dietary cholesterol was thought to be the cause of heart disease, today, science indicates that dietary cholesterol has only a "modest effect on the amount of cholesterol in the bloodstream." The American Heart Association has issued an even stronger statement that there is no link between dietary cholesterol and cardiovascular disease.

BROCCOLI SPROUTS

Broccoli sprouts have been researched extensively and one study conducted by Johns Hopkins University found that the sprouts contain a compound called sulforaphane which has endless benefits. Some of the amazing benefits of sulforaphane include turning on the Nrf2 pathway, which controls over 200 genes; activating the body's endogenous antioxidants; lowering inflammation; assisting in liver detoxification; and slowing the aging process. This same compound exists in broccoli but at a lower amount and you would have to consume more broccoli than palatable to match the benefit of eating a couple of ounces of broccoli sprouts.

OTHER HEALTHY FOOD CHOICES

Celery is filled with phytonutrients that are antioxidants and anti-inflammatory. It is filled with important minerals like iron, zinc, copper, magnesium, calcium, potassium, and selenium. Cabbage is another great choice as it has been shown to contain compounds that improve heart health, improve digestive health, and reduce the risk of certain cancers. These compounds are a type of flavonoid called anthocyanins and are prevalent in red cabbage. Blueberries are another food that contains anthocyanins as well as anthocyanidins. These compounds have been found to positively affect endothelial function and lower blood pressure, along with other decreasing risk factors for heart disease. While fresh organic blueberries can be expensive, frozen organic blueberries are a perfectly healthy alternative.

Mushrooms are known to be an excellent choice to eat. They stimulate the immune system, have antitumor properties, are a source of Vitamin D, and help ameliorate metabolic syndrome. Nuts are a terrific source of healthy fats if you don't eat too many. Walnuts have been studied extensively and found to benefit brain health, heart health, and offer cancer prevention. Nuts are one of the foods that need to be organic. They are very susceptible to pests and are heavily sprayed with pesticides. Nuts are also subject to mycotoxins depending upon how they are stored. Peanuts are quite vulnerable to mold, so one should be cautious about their consumption.

Radishes contain phytochemicals called isothiocyanates and are associated with the inhibition of several cancers. These isothiocyanates protect against DNA damage, inhibit tumor formation, and trigger apoptosis. Apoptosis is defined as a form of programmed cell death. While this sounds particularly bad, it is a normal and genetically regulated process. Green tea has long been touted for its health benefits. It is due to a particular type of polyphenol called catechins. The most beneficial of all of these catechins is called epigallocatechin gallate (EGCG). The list of benefits found in EGCG includes killing cancer cells, stopping cancer growth, blocking cancer activation, improved blood sugar control, and a reduced risk of cardiovascular disease.

There are thousands of phytochemicals that have great health benefits. They are not limited to fruits and vegetables but are also found in nuts, seeds, whole grains, legumes, tea, coffee, herbs, and spices. Some of the known benefits of herbs and spices include the positive effect of sage on cognition, the inhibition of free radicals by rosemary, the removal of heavy metals by cilantro, the anti-nausea properties of mint and ginger, the antioxidant and antibacterial effects of basil and parsley, the antifungal properties of clove, the antiviral and antibacterial effects of lemon, the antiviral properties of coconut oil, and the antifungal effect of cinnamon.

AMINO ACIDS IN FOODS

Methionine and glycine are two amino acids found in foods that have important health benefits. We need these amino acids to protect our tissues and to prevent diseases like diabetes, heart disease, stroke, and cancer. Methionine lowers the risk of fatty liver disease as well as the risks of depression and anxiety. Glycine stabilizes blood sugar, promotes quality sleep, and protects our skin and bones. Once again, the need for balance is clear with these two important amino acids. Too little of either of them leads to health issues and so does an excess of either of them.

How you prepare your food and the tools that you use can be as important as what you eat. It is ill advised to cook, heat, or store food in plastic or Styrofoam containers. Avoid drinking or storing water or other liquids in plastic bottles because plastic is a known endocrine disrupter. Use glass instead. Avoid using aluminum foil or pots and pans with aluminum. There are great alternatives like parchment paper and pots made from ceramic, glass, and cast iron. Some stainless-steel pots can leach nickel at high heat so invest in brands like HOMICHEF and Jarhill, which are nickel free. If possible, reduce your purchases of canned foods. While there are claims that the harmful BPA has been removed from the lining of cans, the replacement chemical is equally as harmful.

It takes time, money, creativity, and effort to prepare healthy meals, but there is a no more important task. Chronic disease accounts for 1.7 million American deaths every year.

According to the CDC, 70 percent of health-care costs in the US are due to lifestyle and are preventable. Health care is one of the country's largest industries. The costs associated with health

> The way we produce food through industrialized agriculture and the way that we consume food in the US is responsible for the widespread amount of chronic disease in this country. We need to consider the social determinants of health and drastically improve the access to health care and healthy food for all people. It is criminal that in a country of such abundance, people lack access to healthy food.

care have increased faster than the median annual income. While multiple factors are contributing to this meteoric rise, preventable chronic disease is the main factor. A study titled "An Unhealthy America: The Economic Burden of Chronic Disease—Charting a New Course to Save Lives and Increase Productivity and Economic Growth" by Ross Devol and Armen Bedroussian was completed for the Milken Institute, a nonpartisan think tank. The study concluded that chronic disease costs the US economy nearly $1.3 trillion annually. This includes not only the costs of treatment of chronic disease but also costs associated with the loss of productivity in the workplace. Perhaps medical schools should consider increasing the amount of education devoted to nutrition. Currently, it is shockingly deficient. I think people must take charge of their health and become their own health advocate, but it would be helpful for doctors dispensing care and advice to have a greater knowledge of nutrition. Even things as simple as eating what's in season, eating lots of different colors, avoiding factory-farmed livestock, prioritizing fruits and vegetables, and avoiding chemicals, pesticides, added hormones, antibiotics, and additives in your food, when possible, will all be helpful. Remember, you are what you eat!

FRANK'S STORY

As an example of how lifestyle, particularly nutrition choices, can impact disease and its treatment and prevention, I want to share a story I heard about a man who was a cook in the Navy. After more than thirty years of cooking for sailors and eating the same food, Frank became overweight, diabetic, and ultimately had a heart attack. When he first started cooking on the ship, he did so in a relatively healthy manner using fresh, whole foods in the preparation of the meals. After a while, the military chose to purchase complete meals in packages. These packaged meals were made from high-fat, high-salt, high-calorie, cheap, processed foods. They were referred to as "industrial food" and paved the way for what we now know as "fast food." The food industry, the agricultural industry and the chemical industry joined forces to create abundance in the food supply. While this endeavor did address food insecurity and offer convenience and extend shelf life of food, it came at a high cost to our health. Food production output has been maximized at the expense of nutritional value. As a result of this widespread consumption of fast food, by 2008, nearly 30 percent of people wanting to enlist in the military failed to meet the minimum standards for height, weight, and fitness. Frank was not alone in dealing with serious health issues. It turns out that quite a few retired servicepeople suffer from diabetes, cardiovascular disease, and high blood pressure. These issues were directly correlated with their lifestyle choices and, specifically, their nutrition.

As Frank began to recover from his heart attack, he decided to completely alter his eating and cooking habits. He committed to focusing exclusively on fresh, whole foods. No more fast or industrial food! Six months after Frank began his healthy new eating and cooking habits, he lost sixty pounds, lowered his blood pressure dramatically, and improved his glucose numbers to the point where he no longer was diabetic. He recounts that changing his habits was not an easy task but feels that the difficulty was well worth the improvement in his health.

ACTION STEPS

➤ Consider reducing your caloric intake—moderately, not drastically.

➤ If you can't identify symptoms that you are experiencing, try an elimination diet to determine if there is a particular food responsible for your symptoms.

➤ Instead of following a specific diet for a short while, adopt a lifestyle of healthy eating habits for the long term.

➤ Familiarize yourself with the ingredients on food labels.

➤ Consume only wild-caught fish.

➤ Cut down or eliminate sugar.

➤ Avoid processed seed oils like the plague.

CHAPTER 8

MOVEMENT:
You Don't Need to Be an
Endurance Athlete

UNLIKE OUR ANCESTORS, THE AVERAGE person today is sedentary for about nine to ten hours a day and that's not counting time sleeping. Physical activity has decreased a great deal in large part due to advances in automation, transportation, and technology. At a time when people had to do laundry by hand, more energy was exerted. Before the automotive industry exploded, people walked most places or at least had to walk to get to the available modes of transportation. We all know that the ubiquitous use of the computer has resulted in people sitting at their desks for hours at a time, day after day. Today, the amount of time spent standing, walking, and exerting energy has decreased by a dramatic amount.

LOSS OF MUSCLE MASS

Muscles are constantly changing from cycles of breakdown, which is called catabolism, and from cycles of restoration, which is called anabolism. As we age, the formation of new muscle declines as the

breakdown of muscle continues without slowing down. The
reduction in our mitochondria
also contributes to sarcopenia.
Additional adverse effects of a
decline in muscle mass are the
increase in chronic inflammation
and the increase in frailty and
susceptibility to falling.

> The dangers of today's
> inactivity are profound
> and abundant. One of
> the main consequences of
> inactivity is muscle loss.
> As we age, this begins to
> happen around our forties
> and it is called sarcopenia.

CARDIOVASCULAR BENEFITS

Lack of exercise or inactivity can increase the risk of hypertension
or high blood pressure, which in turn increases the risk of stroke
or kidney disease. Exercise makes the heart stronger so it can pump
blood more efficiently and lower this risk. Poor coronary blood flow
and increased LDL cholesterol levels are also associated with a sedentary lifestyle, and they contribute to an increased risk of developing cardiovascular disease. As we age and as we become less active,
our bones become weak, and we can develop osteoporosis which
can lead to bone fractures. Certain cancers such as colon and breast
cancer are on the list of the consequences of inactivity. Being active
results in the greater efficiency of the colon moving waste through
the body and decreases the time of potential carcinogens lurking in
our body. As inactivity increases, the metabolism functions less optimally, and type 2 diabetes and obesity risks increase. Certain neurotransmitters which regulate mood are activated with exercise, and
inactivity increases the risk of anxiety and depression. Finally, lack
of movement can adversely affect our immune system as well as the
necessary balance of hormones.

HEIDI'S STORY

A friend of mine named Heidi told me about how exercise had a transformational impact on her life. She is in her early fifties and always hated any form of exercise. Her diet consisted of fried chicken tenders, doughnuts, and sugar-filled soda. This explained, at least in part, why she weighed two hundred eighty pounds. One day, Heidi realized that she had to make some dramatic changes to her lifestyle if she wanted to be around for her children. She radically altered her diet and promptly lost forty-two pounds. Delighted with her progress, she became inspired to be disciplined about her food choices. Then, without any warning, Heidi hit a weight-loss plateau. The scale would not budge. Discouraged, she searched for her next course correct and accepted that, after a lifetime of being sedentary, it was time to get moving!

Heidi found the thought of an exercise routine to be daunting. Not only had she strenuously avoided any kind of movement for most of her life, but she also found the logistics of adding one more thing to her schedule to be overwhelming. She wondered how much time she would need to exercise. How would she fit it into her already busy daily schedule? Should she join a gym or download an app or try an online exercise website? Finally, Heidi just decided to take a walk outside around the block. That first walk led to a longer walk and then running for half of the duration of the walk. Eventually, Heidi was running 5Ks, then 10Ks, and even a half-marathon. Not only did she lose one hundred pounds, her struggle with anxiety and depression vastly improved. For the first time in years, Heidi had confidence and self-esteem.

I am not suggesting that everyone should take up running. I am, however, suggesting that everyone should try to incorporate some form of movement into their life. Figure out which type of exercise you like. That will be the kind with which you will stick. Try rock climbing, dancing, martial arts, or anything to begin your new routine. When done consistently, over time, you'll establish a routine, and it will be easy to continue. The return on this investment into your health will be profound. At the very least, you will be happier, healthier, and, hopefully, you will live longer!

DIFFERENT FORMS OF EXERCISE

While there are many different types of exercise, the ones which will receive the most attention in this chapter are resistance training, cardiovascular training, and high-intensity interval training. There is a constant debate as to which type of exercise is best to do, but the reality is that each one has distinct benefits, and the most optimum outcome will result from doing a variety of all three types.

CARDIOVASCULAR TRAINING

The first type is cardiovascular training, also known as aerobic exercise. This type can vary in intensity from low to high but is described as using oxygen for energy. Cardio, as it is called, is best for losing body fat if you consistently do some form of this exercise an average of 120 minutes a week. This is because cardio causes an elevation in your heart rate, and that triggers a higher calorie burn. Because exercise increases heart rate and both blood flow and oxygen to the brain, cognitive function improves.[102] The types of exercise that qualify as cardio include jumping rope, running, jogging, swimming, using elliptical machines, stationary bikes, and taking classes that involve exercise which raises your heart rate. The benefits of this exercise include strengthening of the heart, an increase in muscle endurance and capillary size, and an overall increased efficiency of blood flow. Specific types of aerobic exercise are running, jogging, biking, swimming, skating, and rowing. The number of calories that you burn depends on the intensity of the exercise and your body size.

RESISTANCE TRAINING

The second type of exercise is resistance training, also known as weight training. The distinct benefits of this are building muscle, decreasing the risk of osteoporosis, and improving metabolism. This is an anaerobic activity that breaks down glucose for energy instead of oxygen. Glucose is used through a process called glycolysis. It is a quick production of energy and produces lactic acid which can make your muscles sore. There are several ways to achieve resistance training. You can use resistance bands, which are like giant rubber bands which provide resistance when stretched and are easy to travel with due to their portability. You can use weight machines, free weights such as kettlebells, dumbbells, barbells, and weighted balls. There is also suspension equipment, which utilizes gravity along with the user's body weight, and simply using one's own body weight doing exercises like squats, push-ups, and planks. The degree of progress depends upon the number of sets, the number of repetitions, the size of the weights used, and the frequency with which one trains. The benefits of this type of exercise include improvement and maintenance of muscle mass, endurance and strength, protection from injuries, increased balance and flexibility, weight management, reduced risk of chronic disease, improved sleep and cognition, and increased bone density, which reduces the risk of fractures.[103] One interesting thing that should be noted is that the more muscle that you have, the greater your "resting metabolism" is. This translates into the number of calories that you burn while resting. Weight training increases your caloric burn in the hours following a resistance workout at a higher rate than after doing a cardiovascular workout.

HIGH-INTENSITY INTERVAL TRAINING

The third type of exercise that you should have in your routine is called high-intensity interval training, or HIIT. This form of exercise is ideal for people who have time constraints as it involves short bursts of intense exercise followed by lengthy periods of low-intensity exercise. You can achieve terrific results in doing twenty minutes of HIIT, and you can burn a lot of calories in a short amount of time. This type of exercise improves cardiorespiratory and metabolic health, reduces body fat, improves mental health, lowers blood pressure, lowers stress, improves sleep, and even reduces joint stiffness.

There is growing research suggesting that HIIT may have better results than moderate-intensity and longer-duration, or what is referred to as "steady state," exercise.[104] One of the advantages of this type of exercise is that you don't need any kind of equipment. You can achieve beneficial results by applying the method to swimming, running, biking, and even walking. Ideally, you should use a one-to-two interval, or thirty seconds of intense exercise followed by sixty seconds of less-intense exercise. A study found that HIIT can increase the length of your telomeres and help you age more optimally. Telomeres are the caps at the end of each strand of DNA that protect our chromosomes.[105] When trying to decide which type of exercise is best for you, keep in mind that a range of many types of exercise is best. Your muscles adapt to the same form of exercise if done to the exclusion of other types. Ideally, you should do a bit of each of the exercises described for optimal results.

On the other hand, it should be noted that a March 2021 study conducted in Sweden suggested that HIIT may have unexpected drawbacks.[106] The study advises that the benefits of extremely vigorous exercise may depend on how much exercise one is doing. It was concluded that excessive exercise training can substantially impair one's mitochondria, which is the opposite effect desired from exercise. Ideally, we all want more mitochondria as they are thought to contribute to better cellular and metabolic health. While the study was relatively small, it's a reminder that exercise affects your biology on a cellular level. We know that the muscles of those who exercise have more mitochondria than those who neglect exercise. The research into longevity reveals that the quality and quantity of one's mitochondria acutely impact longevity.

NON-EXERCISE ACTIVITY THERMOGENESIS

An overlooked factor that can positively affect your metabolic rate is something called non-exercise activity thermogenesis, or NEAT. This is associated with your resting metabolic rate, which is a measure of how many calories you expend while breathing, resting, sleeping, eating, and doing gentle activities.

NEAT is affected by activities like cooking, house cleaning, gardening, shopping, climbing stairs, and even fidgeting. The number of calories burned by NEAT varies from individual to individual depending upon body size and genetics. It can even vary between two people of the same size. It turns out that this type of light movement plays an important role in your overall health. When combined with an intentional exercise routine, NEAT contributes to an optimal result.

As a matter of fact, several studies are suggesting that a daily hour of intense exercise followed by eight to ten hours of sitting does not yield good results and can promote weight gain. A study completed by John D. Akins concluded that sitting around after a workout can negate any metabolic benefits that you gained from the workout.

The study followed one group of people who spent four days of prolonged sitting without any exercise and another group of people who spent four days of sitting with one hour spent on the treadmill. There was no difference found in the two groups in terms of lipid, glucose, or insulin metabolism. Sitting for excessive amounts of time renders the body resistant to a daily hour of exercise. "People seem to become resistant to the normal metabolic benefits of acute aerobic exercise after prolonged inactivity."[107] It turns out that, as they say, sitting really is the new smoking!

COGNITIVE FUNCTION IMPROVEMENT

For many years, it was thought aerobic exercise is the best for brain health, but in recent years, resistance training and even low-intensity exercise have been shown to improve cognitive function. Exercise causes a surge in the brain of neurotransmitters dopamine, norepinephrine, and serotonin, which are required for neurogenesis (the growth of new neurons).

Studies have shown that exercise increases hippocampal volume and creates and maintains brain cells. Also produced from exercise are neurotrophins, which lead to greater brain plasticity.

Fasting is another effective means to stimulate BDNF, and I will discuss that in chapter 14. Like so many other aspects of our biology, BDNF declines as we age. Declining levels of this critical protein have been connected to depression, anxiety, memory decline, and neurodegenerative diseases. The current belief is that resistance training and even yoga and tai chi, in addition to aerobic activity, all stimulate BDNF. This supports the old adage that "a healthy body leads to a healthy mind."

> Another critical benefit of exercise is the production of brain-derived neurotrophic factor, known as BDNF. BDNF is a protein found in the hippocampus part of your brain that is involved with neuroplasticity and both promotes and maintains brain function by maintaining existing brain cells and growing new neurons.

Some people focus on quadrupedal movements. These involve moving on all fours (hands and feet) and are said to have neuromuscular benefits. Research shows that these types of movements help with memory and spatial awareness as well as being good for coordination and core strength.

MOLECULAR RESPONSE TO EXERCISE

A recent study from Stanford University brings us a little bit closer to developing a simple blood test to determine one's physical fitness. The study researched the molecular responses to acute exercise. It was considered to be a small-participant study as it had only thirty-six subjects, between the ages of forty to seventy-five, each representing a range of health and fitness. The researchers drew blood at two, fifteen, thirty, and sixty minutes after a ten-minute intense run on a treadmill. The scientists were quite surprised to find a substantial change in the subject's molecular profiles from only ten minutes of acute exercise. The study concluded that acute physical activity leads to several changes in metabolic, cardiovascular, and immune pathways. The co-author of the study, Kévin Contrepois, PhD, stated that "aerobic fitness is one of the best measures of longevity, so a simple blood test that can provide that information would be valuable to personal health monitoring."[108]

BENEFITS OF EXERCISE

As I have discussed, the benefits of exercise are endless. Many consider it to be the most transformative thing you can do for your brain because of its immediate effects. Not only do you feel great after exercise, but your focus and attention are heightened for hours afterward. While some of the immediate effects are transient, they begin to last for a longer time with a consistent routine of exercise. Your reaction time improves. Your energy increases. Your immune system strengthens. Your deep sleep increases, and due to the increase in neurotransmitters like dopamine, serotonin, and noradrenaline, your mood elevates. This release of neurotransmitters is protective for the brain. Your prefrontal cortex and hippocampus become stronger, which is essential as they are most vulnerable to neurodegenerative disease. Additional benefits include the increased blood flow to the brain, supplying it with oxygen and glucose; the maintenance and improvement of your stability, balance, mobility, flexibility, and strength (both physical and mental); and improvement to one's endurance and circulatory system.

While there is much debate among exercise professionals as to the balance of aerobic and resistance training and the appropriate degree of duration and intensity, there is universal agreement as to the harms associated with overtraining. Overexercising can result in impaired sleep, hormonal imbalance, increased injuries, a rise in cortisol levels, and inflammation. I really wish I had known this years ago as I ran six to seven days a week for about thirty years and now have two chronically sore, arthritic knees. It turns out that diversity of exercise is quite beneficial. Not only will changing when you work out, which tools you use during your workout, and what types of exercise you do to avoid the dreaded body adaptation, resulting in less progress, but you will reduce the risk of injuries from repetitive movements. Another important way to reduce the risk of injury is to take time to learn about and to master the correct form for any activity.

DON'T FORGET TO REST AND RECOVER

There is a growing area of exercise science devoted to the physiology of rest, recovery, and rebuilding. Olympic and high-level athletes take this very seriously for both optimal performance and reduction in injury risk. Rest is essential for muscle growth and continued progress. Weight training causes microscopic tears in muscles and only during periods of rest do fibroblasts repair these tears. You must prioritize sleep as part of recovery as well as schedule days off and incorporate days of lighter exercise.

GENOMICS AND EXERCISE

An interesting and emerging field is that of genomics and genetic sequencing to determine which exercise-related variants you have. I describe this field in more depth in chapter 16 on genetics, epigenetics, and genomics, and the reality is that, despite the unfounded claims of certain entrepreneurs, science has not evolved sufficiently to determine the best form of exercise according to one's variants. It is known that genes such as FTO, ADRB2, BDNF, ACTN3, NFIA-AS2, ADRB3, NRF2, GSTP1, PGC1a, and COL5A1 are a selection of variants that influence one's response to exercise. They can inform one's propensity for weight loss, enjoyment of exercise, the likelihood of excellence in endurance versus power and strength, propensity for muscle damage, and risk of injury. I am excited to see what the future brings in terms of genomics and guidance for which exercise is the most appropriate for our individuality.

BEST TIME TO EXERCISE

Studies have shown that exercising in a fasted state (in other words, before breakfast) can result in better outcomes as well as walking after dinner or any meal can assist in the digestive process. Ideally, you just want to maintain some sort of movement throughout the day. If your work requires sitting for long periods of time, try to commit to getting up every forty-five minutes and walking around or moving in some way. There are many tracking devices to encourage you to maintain a consistent routine of movement. These include smart-phone apps, Fitbits, or the Ōura Ring which, among other things, track your activity level every day. These devices help you to learn about your health and assist in the valuable accumulation of data. You can use this data to inform your plan going forward.

> Regarding the best time to exercise, the best time is when you can do it consistently. When people ask this question, it makes me think of the Chinese proverb: "The best time to plant a tree is twenty years ago. The second best time is now."

Everyone can and will benefit from incorporating some sort of movement or exercise into their daily routine. People in their eighties and beyond can adapt to an exercise routine even if they haven't been previously active. Start *today*. Start simply and slowly and make it a way of life.

ACTION STEPS

➢ If you are just beginning to incorporate exercise into your life, start slow.

➢ Figure out which type of movement you prefer and make it a part of your daily routine.

➢ Listen to music or exercise with a friend. Both can increase enjoyment.

➢ Do not overdo it. Always build in time to rest and recover.

➢ Create a mental state which will allow you to be consistent. Find your motivation.

➢ Take note of the many benefits including improved sleep, improved mental as well as physical well-being, improved metabolism, and increased endurance and muscle mass.

CHAPTER 9

RESPIRATORY PHYSIOLOGY:
Also Known as Breathing

I REALIZE THAT IT MAY seem odd to devote a chapter, or any discussion at all, to breathing. Most of us believe that breathing is something that we do automatically and is low on our list of things to improve. It turns out that how we breathe is as important as what we eat, how we exercise, and our sleep quality. How we breathe has a direct impact on our physiology and overall health. Traditionally, breath work has been the domain of yoga and meditation, but it is now becoming more of a focus of health as more studies reveal the association between proper breathing and stress reduction, increased focus, better endurance, better endocrine health, better heart health, better brain health, and improved sleep quality. Controlled breathing helps lower your heart rate and blood pressure, improve your immune system, and balance carbon dioxide and oxygen blood levels. Research reveals that proper breathing has been studied throughout history by many different cultures. I have read that over 80 percent of the population breathes improperly.

THE PHYSIOLOGY OF BREATHING

Respiration is the metabolic process of oxygen intake and carbon dioxide release. When we are born, our autonomic nervous system triggers optimally functional breathing through our nose as our diaphragm expands and retracts. The diaphragm is a muscle at the base of the lungs. When you inhale, your diaphragm contracts and moves downward thereby allowing expansion of the lungs. When you exhale, your diaphragm expands and moves upward.

The respiratory rate is the number of breaths a person takes. It is measured per minute, and the average is twelve to eighteen breaths per minute which translates to about 18,000 to 25,000 breaths per twenty-four-hour period.

The respiratory rate reflects the connection between the brain and the levels of oxygen and carbon dioxide in the blood. When either oxygen in the blood is low or carbon dioxide is too high, the brain sends a message to increase the number of breaths. Different variations of respiratory rate include bradypnea, which is decreased respiratory rate; tachypnea, which is elevated respiratory rate due to shallow breathing; dyspnea, which refers to shortness of breath due to elevated, normal, or decreased respiratory rate; hyperpnea, which is abnormally deep breathing; and apnea, which is the absence of breath.

BREATHING BECOMES MORE DIFFICULT AS WE AGE

The dismal reality is that lung function declines as we age, and our lung capacity diminishes. This decline begins at around the age of thirty-five. The process of decline begins with the absorption of less oxygen as we breathe and retention of more residual air in our lungs. The trachea (windpipe) increases in size, and as our breathing capacity declines, the ability of our lungs to fight infection diminishes. As we become more sedentary, our diaphragm weakens. This is relevant because optimal breathing takes place using the diaphragm. Diaphragmatic breathing is referred to as belly breathing and maintains the proper balance of oxygen and carbon dioxide in our blood and slows our heart rate and lowers blood pressure. When we inhale, we draw in oxygen (O_2) and when we exhale, we release carbon dioxide (CO_2). It is critical for these to be in balance.

NOSE BREATHING VS. MOUTH BREATHING

> Breathing through the mouth rather than the nose is an indicator of breathing dysfunction.

To employ belly breathing or diaphragmatic breathing, one must breathe through their nose. While breathing through the nose helps to retain moisture in the body and reduce dehydration, it sterilizes and moistens the air before it reaches the lungs, increases the delivery of nitric oxide, and improves immune response. It is truly fundamental to optimal health as it filters the amount of oxygen that the body needs and helps to maintain the critical balance between oxygen and carbon dioxide. This contributes to a reduction in anxiety, asthma, and an increase in sleep quality and overall performance.

THE BOHR EFFECT

In 1904, a Danish physiologist named Christian Bohr discovered what is today called the Bohr effect. This phenomenon is when you breathe through your mouth, you expel too much carbon dioxide and less oxygen is released from hemoglobin into your cells. This results in lowered blood oxygen and less blood flow to your organs. Breathing through the mouth causes breathing from the chest and is much shallower than when breathing through the nose. Mouth breathers tend to have poor ventilation and perfusion which affects the total volume of blood and air reaching the pulmonary capillaries. Even though one breathes more air when breathing through the mouth, there is less oxygen uptake in the blood, resulting in lower oxygen saturation. This means that there is less oxygen delivered to the cells. In addition to the potential for neurological issues, mouth breathing is associated with snoring, obstructive sleep apnea, dental issues, and a host of other health conditions. It is well documented that mouth breathing has led to an evolutionary change in facial structure. Biological anthropologists have discovered that both airways and jaws are now smaller, leaving less room for teeth. Faces are longer and narrower, and jaws are less prominent. These facial structural changes are thought to account for the increasing number of obstructive sleep apnea cases.

DYSFUNCTIONAL BREATHING

The optimal number of breaths you should take in one day is between eighteen thousand and twenty-five thousand. Most people overbreathe to the degree of nearly double the number of optimal breaths. Overbreathing can quickly become hyperventilating. The symptoms of hyperventilating are quick, shallow breaths. This causes a "decrease in carbon dioxide," pressure in the alveoli (our lungs) and arteries, an "increase in arterial pH (respiratory alkalosis)," "constriction of cerebral arteries," and "increased production of lactic and pyruvic acid." We are not aware of it when it is chronic "hyperventilation syndrome."[109] This syndrome is common and occurs when you appear to be breathing normally, but are, in fact, inhaling too much air. This habit keeps carbon dioxide levels in the blood too low and disrupts oxygen homeostasis. This chronic overbreathing adversely affects the autonomic nervous system, heart rate, and blood pressure. Short breaths trigger the release of cortisol and adrenaline. When these stress hormones are released, our autonomic nervous system shifts from parasympathetic mode to sympathetic mode. The parasympathetic nervous system is referred to as the "rest and digest" mode and is responsible for relaxation and slowing the heart rate. The sympathetic nervous system is referred to as the "fight or flight" mode and is responsible for an increase in heart rate and several other stress responses.[110] The harder you breathe, the more your blood vessels constrict, and the less oxygen is delivered to your cells. We have between sixty thousand to one hundred thousand (depending upon which source you trust) miles of blood vessels throughout the body, and whether they are constricted or dilated depends on your breath. Andrew Huberman, PhD, a neuroscientist, emphasizes that many of us suffer from autonomic dysregulation. To feel and perform our best, we must learn how to regulate our nervous system. The first step is efficient breathing.

FORMS OF RESPIRATORY ACTION

365 METHOD

You can choose to breathe fast or slow, shallow or deep. There are many studied methods of improving one's breathing technique. The common goal of these different techniques is to increase blood flow to the brain, increase overall circulation, and improve comprehensive efficiency. The first of these techniques is called the 365 method or what is also known as "cardiac coherence." For hundreds of years, the connection between respiration and the cardiovascular system has been studied. This method, which is based on the interaction between slow, deep breathing and the vagus nerve, aligns one's breathing with their heart rate. The vagus nerve is the tenth (and longest and most complex) of the twelve pairs of cranial nerves beginning in the brain. This nerve is responsible for all communications between the brain and the other internal organs. When the vagus nerve is stimulated, one's heart rate and blood pressure both decrease, muscles relax, and a sense of calm occurs. This method is known as the 365 method because it is to be practiced every day. One should spend five minutes inhaling in for five seconds and exhaling for five seconds. In a five-minute period, there should be six cycles of this breathing. The five-minute sequence should be repeated three times a day.

4-7-8 METHOD

The next technique is called the 4-7-8 method or the "relaxing breath," and while there are not many scientific studies on this method, there is plenty of anecdotal evidence of its efficacy. It is both recommended and taught by Dr. Andrew Weil and is done by inhaling through the nose for a count of four, holding the breath for a count of seven, and exhaling through the mouth for a count of eight. One should repeat each cycle of this breathing four times in a row. The result will be reduced anxiety, reduced anger response, improved sleep, and overall relaxation.

PRANAYAMA BREATHING

Pranayama breathing is also known as "yogic breathing" and is an important part of yoga practice. In Sanskrit, the word *prana* means life force, and the word *ayama* means extending or stretching. There are many types of this breathing that are based on controlling one's breath and, depending upon which type, can result in an increase of energy stress reduction.

ALTERNATE NOSTRIL BREATHING

Alternate nostril breathing is one type that lowers your pulse, reduces your blood pressure, and can even increase your cognitive abilities. To put this into practice, use your right thumb to close your right nostril leaving you to breathe through your left nostril. Then do the same switching your thumb to the left side and breathing through your right nostril. Continue back and forth with this process for about five minutes. The right nostril activates the sympathetic nervous system and the left hemisphere of the brain. Breathing through the left nostril activates the parasympathetic nervous system and the right hemisphere of the brain.

BOX BREATHING

Box breathing, also known as "Navy SEAL" or "tactical breathing," is a technique used by athletes, police officers, nurses, and others to calm oneself, increase focus, and for respiratory strengthening. To try this method, inhale through the nose for a count of four seconds, hold the breath for four seconds, exhale through the mouth for four seconds and finally, hold the breath again for another four seconds. Repeat this sequence several times a day.

BUTEYKO BREATHING

Buteyko breathing is a technique named for a Ukrainian doctor who used the technique as a treatment for asthma and other respiratory conditions. Dr. Buteyko was convinced that improper breathing posed a greater risk to one's health than poor eating and drinking. His method is an antidote to overbreathing and is based on slow, nasal breathing. His theory is that when breathing is deliberate, the heart rate will slow and oxygen will be utilized more efficiently. One should aim to take fewer, lighter breaths. It is a misconception that deep breaths are best to achieve a calm state. In fact, deep breaths encourage overbreathing. To use this method of breathing, one first must determine their "controlled pause," which is the length of time after exhalation until the experience of a slight urge to take another breath.

The objective is to increase your breath holding or controlled pause. To give you an idea of what the results of this controlled pause test mean, here are some metrics: If you are only able to hold your breath for ten seconds or less, you have a "serious" breathing disability which will soon result in chronic health issues. If you can hold your breath for ten to twenty seconds, you are considered to have a "significant" breathing disability that is worthy of attention. If you can hold your breath for twenty to forty seconds, you fall into the category of most adults and have a "mild" level of reduced breathing capacity. If you can hold your breath for forty to sixty seconds,

This "controlled pause" reveals your carbon dioxide tolerance. One can measure this by inhaling and exhaling gently and then pinching their nose shut while watching a stopwatch. The number of seconds which pass until the urge to take a breath represents your controlled pause or how long you can comfortably hold your breath. After measuring for this number in seconds, inhale gently, without moving your chest or shoulders, and exhale. Hold your nose for the amount of time your measurement revealed and then breathe normally for one minute. During this one-minute interval, relax and then repeat the process.

you have achieved a high level of respiratory fitness and have accomplished the goal of optimal breathing. Before becoming too discouraged with your results of this test, please know that breathing is something that can be improved with consistent practice. Patrick McKeown, who has written several books about breathing, is a certified Buteyko breathing consultant and credits the method with improving his health.

WIM HOF METHOD

Wim Hof is a Dutch athlete and a unique individual. He is referred to as "The Iceman" and is known for completing extreme endeavors such as swimming underneath ice, climbing Mount Everest in shorts, and running half-marathons in the snow while barefoot. I heard him speak at a conference and have never experienced anything like his presentation. He told us that his grief resulting from his first wife's suicide was responsible for his pursuit of extreme athletics. He is known for his high performance in extremely cold temperatures and is studied mostly for his cold exposure. He attributes his high performance to his breathing method and is a proponent of respiratory control. Hof believes that his method will contribute to your overall resilience. At first glance, one would probably think this is pseudoscience, but Hof and his techniques are the subjects of many university studies.[111] Radboud University Medical Center in the Netherlands, Wayne State University, and the University of California, San Francisco have all conducted several studies and have tested Hof's blood before and after his exercises and found positive results. It appears as if Hof has discovered a method for intentionally controlling one's autonomic nervous and immune systems. This has enormous implications for the pursuit of stress resilience, which is critical to optimal health. According to the Wim Hof Method website, the benefits gained from consistently practicing his methods include increased energy, reduced stress, better sleep, increased focus, improved athletic performance, increased willpower, greater cold tolerance, faster recovery, enhanced creativity, and a stronger immune system. Given that list of incentives, it seems as though it is worth exploring. This technique is quite a bit different than the others referenced in this chapter. Rather than lay out the technique, I am going to refer you to his website, www.wimhofmethod.com, or the internet where many videos lead one through the steps involved in this breathing method. Please note that this type of breathing is not for everyone and is contraindicated for many. This type of breathing, while done by biohackers regularly, can result in ischemia, which is an insufficient blood supply due to an obstruction of blood flow. It is thought to be most useful when enduring cold thermogenesis.

PHYSIOLOGICAL SIGH

This type of breathing is quite interesting. For ages, breathing was believed to be simply a mechanism to provide you with oxygen and to dispel carbon dioxide. As of late, it is understood that it's far more complex than that. Breathing is also a mechanism to control the state of your brain and emotions. A "physiological sigh" is two distinct deep breaths that are twice the volume of a normal breath, followed by an extended exhale. According to Silvia Pagliardini, an associate professor in the Department of Physiology at the University of Alberta, "sighs keep the tiny air sacs in the lungs, the alveoli, from collapsing, and maintain the exchange of oxygen and carbon dioxide." A complete lack of sighing would prevent the alveoli from reopening and would result in hypoxia (a deficiency of oxygen reaching the body's tissues) and death.[112]

Elke Vlemincx, an assistant professor at the Department of Health Sciences at the Vrije Universiteit, has researched the physiology, as well as the psychophysiology, of the sigh. She focused on this form of respiration. Vlemincx found that sighs serve as a homeostatic mechanism for your breathing and emotions.

They can occur during both good and bad emotional states to restore balance. While sighing appears to be essential to well-be-

> A sigh can restore calm and provide relief during periods of stress. It is the quickest, non-pharmaceutical way to downregulate your autonomic nervous system.

ing, excessive amounts of sighing can lead to hyperventilating and is discouraged.[113]

MAXIMUM EXHALE IS KEY

In the mid-1900s, an American choral conductor named Carl Stough became interested in the mechanisms of breathing. When he first began his research, he focused on the relationship between breathing and singing. He later became a "breathing specialist," and in addition to applying his knowledge of breathing to singers, he also applied it to emphysema patients and Olympic athletes, thus confirming the benefits of optimal breathing to everyone. His concept is called "Breathing Coordination" and is based on the findings that one should execute a maximum exhale to maintain a low residual amount of carbon dioxide and to strengthen the diaphragm. Stough felt strongly that the respiratory system is designed to function at maximum efficiency with minimum effort.

IF YOU LEARN TO BREATHE, YOU CAN MASTER ANYTHING

The journalist James Nestor's most recent book is called *Breath* and, as you can probably guess, it's all about breathing. Nestor points out the interesting fact that most prayers share the same respiration rate as optimal breathing. This rate is a five-to-six-second inhale and a five-to-six-second exhale. He states that doing this kind of breathing five minutes a day will lead to healing and he further states fifteen minutes of this breathing every day can improve your metabolism and resolve autoimmune and other chronic diseases. He points out that optimal breathing is not a novel concept, but in the film *American Sniper*, there is a line that states, "If you learn to breathe, you can master anything." Nestor did some self-experimentation and taped his nose for ten days to examine the results of mouth breathing. He found several negative consequences from mouth breathing including snoring and sleep apnea.

Some easy tricks to improve one's breathing while sleeping includes taping one's mouth. I realize that it sounds rather barbaric and probably should not be attempted if you have sinus congestion, but this is a hack done by many biohackers, along with others, trying to improve their breathing while sleeping. Please know that this and all other suggestions should be discussed first with your health-care practitioner. I suspect there are contraindications for who should and who should not attempt this experiment. One should use paper tape (not duct tape or any heavy tape) or the tape made by SomniFix designed especially for this purpose. I have tried it personally and I found that it vastly improved my heart rate variability (HRV) score which is something that I will go into in another chapter. You can also sleep on your side instead of your back or stomach for better breathing and you can lift the portion of your bed where your head rests up five to seven degrees.

WILL'S STORY

My youngest son told me for years about his difficulty getting a good night's sleep. He would wake up feeling tired and remained a bit groggy throughout the day. We tried changing all sorts of different things to improve his sleep habits. It wasn't until I came across studies illustrating the issues associated with mouth breathing that I realized that this could be a cause of his poor sleep. I knew that Will was a mouth breather because his snoring was legendary! When he was about twenty-two years old, we decided to give this experiment a try. We began slowly to avoid discomfort. Will started by wearing the tape during the day for short periods of time to get used to it. He didn't like it at first because it felt strange. It took some time to get used to but, eventually, he trained himself to stop mouth breathing, stop snoring, and switch to nose breathing. His sleep improved massively, and he felt far more energetic and focused throughout the day.

I also shared all that I had learned about the various breathing techniques, and he became enamored of Wim Hof. He began using Wim's techniques and has found many benefits. Along with an overall feeling of well-being, his anxiety has subsided considerably. He feels far more clearheaded, focused, energetic, and balanced due to these lifestyle alterations. Will believes that he has an easier time falling asleep at night and a sense of balance.

The way you breathe has a strong impact on your mitochondria. If you breathe incorrectly, your mitochondria become weak and die off. If you breathe properly, you can enhance your health and performance.

While we tend to take breathing for granted, it is well worth the effort involved to learn breathing techniques because there is a confirmed connection between respiration and optimal health. As you practice these techniques consistently, the breathing center in your brain will be reset. While the various methods described each have different results, the two constants to remember are breathing through your nose instead of your mouth and breathing from your belly instead of your chest. The beauty of focused breathing as a method of healing is that you don't need any special equipment and you can do it almost anywhere, anytime.

ACTION STEPS

➤ Breathe through your nose, not your mouth.

➤ If you are so inclined, try mouth taping (but only after clearing this with your health-care practitioner).

➤ If you snore, do a sleep apnea test.

➤ After experimenting with several different breathing techniques, choose one and do it consistently.

➤ Monitor your respiratory rate with one of the many devices available. Collect your data and adjust accordingly.

➤ Do not try any breathing technique while you are driving or are near water.

CHAPTER 10

HORMONES:
When These Decline, So Do You

IN MY OPINION, HORMONES GET short shrift as to the important role they play in our daily lives. Because they are so powerful, the smallest imbalance can result in serious issues. Women experience unrelenting hormonal fluctuation throughout their life. When hormones become unbalanced, a variety of health issues and an increase in one's risk of disease result.

THE ENDOCRINE SYSTEM

Starting with a little background, the endocrine system is defined as a series of glands in your body that secrete hormones. The eight major glands which make up the endocrine system are located throughout your body. In your brain, there is the hypothalamus, the pituitary gland, and the pineal gland. Moving down toward your neck, you will find the thyroid gland. The thymus gland is in your lungs, the adrenal glands are located on top of your kidneys, and the pancreas is tucked deep inside your body behind your stomach. Your sex glands are in your pelvic region and consist of ovaries if you are a woman and testes if you are a man. These glands secrete hormones that are transported through the bloodstream to various organs and tissues. Hormones are defined as signaling molecules or chemical messengers that regulate physiology and behavior. The main hormones to be concerned with are thyroid, insulin, estrogen, progesterone, prolactin, testosterone, serotonin, cortisol, adrenaline, and growth hormone. The hormones fall into four main chemical classes, which are amino acid derived: eicosanoids derived from lipids, steroid hormones derived from cholesterol, and peptide, polypeptide, and protein hormones.

The endocrine system is involved in the secretion of so many hormones and is so complex that I will refer you to the multitude of books devoted exclusively to the topic. I will, however, cover what you can do to balance your hormones to optimize how you feel and to reduce the risk of disease. The levels, timing, and balance of hormones play a critical role in your body's function and health.

REPLACEMENT THERAPY

The area that I find the most interesting when discussing hormones is the replacement of estrogen, progesterone, and testosterone.

The benefits that were highlighted early in the research include the reduction of menopausal symptoms as well as the significant reduction in risk in many chronic diseases. One of the most well-known studies, the Framingham study, discusses the benefits of estrogen and its protection against cardiovascular disease.[114] Other studies through-

Despite the widespread controversy surrounding hormone replacement therapy (HRT), there is over seventy years' worth of evidence of the benefits of hormone replacement therapy documented in the scientific literature.

out the 1990s revealed that many of the diseases that plague women as they age can be ameliorated by hormone replacement therapy. Things began to get confusing around 2002 when the reports from the Women's Health Initiative were published. This study cost the National Institutes of Health $1 billion and is thought by many to be the most flawed study ever conducted.

It ended earlier than planned because too many of the subjects of the study were getting breast cancer, heart disease, stroke or dementia, or dying. When news of the study hit the press, women and their doctors everywhere were scared away from continuing use of their HRT and abruptly stopped using their prescribed hormones.

SYNTHETIC VS. BIOIDENTICAL HORMONES

Years later and after in-depth analysis, many doctors and scientists have concluded that the study should not be relied upon. Some of the critical components of the study were problematic. To begin, the participants of the study were already past what is now known to be the appropriate window for HRT. Many had already been in menopause for years and it is believed that starting to replace hormones more than eighteen months after menopause presents risks. Secondly, the participants in the study were asked to self-report their symptoms and the existence of any disease. Self-reporting alone is inconclusive at best and downright useless at worst. Third, the subjects of the study were given Premarin and Prempro, both synthetic pharmaceuticals derived from the urine of a pregnant horse. While I do realize that people have pig valves as replacement valves in their hearts and some thyroid medications are derived from pigs, it is worth pondering that the hormone physiology of a horse may not correspond with that of a female human. It is my opinion that using conjugated equine estrogen as hormone replacement is a bad idea. An alternative to synthetic hormone replacement is bioidentical hormone replacement therapy, known as BHRT. Bioidentical hormones have been around since the 1930s. They are compounded in a lab using soy or yams for the basic chemical structure. They are produced to mimic the same structure which makes up natural hormones in the human body. They are defined as having the same molecular structure as a substance produced in the body.

SEX HORMONES

Sex hormones are those which influence reproduction and sexual development, puberty, the promotion of hair growth, inflammatory responses, the distribution of body fat, and the regulation of cholesterol levels.

ESTROGEN

Both men and women have testosterone and estrogen but in different amounts. Estrogen in men is responsible for the maturity of sperm cells, a healthy libido, and the protection of the brain, heart, and bones. While estrogen in men occurs at a much lower level than in women, it increases as men age while their testosterone levels decrease. The key to optimal health is to maintain a balance of one's hormones for both men and women.

While six types of estrogen have been identified, the main three which are dominant during the different phases of a woman's life are estrone (E1), estradiol (E2), and estriol (E3).

Estrone is an intermediate estrogen or a milder form. It is produced in the fatty bodily tissues and becomes more prevalent during menopause. Estradiol is the most active and most powerful estrogen and is dominant from puberty up until menopause. It is produced in the ovaries. The plummeting levels of estradiol which occur at menopause are responsible for hot flashes, night sweats, mood swings, and diminished libido. Estriol is the least powerful form of estrogen, is formed in the liver, and is only dominant during pregnancy. It is thought to have some anticancer properties. All these forms of estrogen enter the cells and then bind to the estrogen receptors. Estrogen receptors are everywhere in the body, including the ovaries, brain, heart, vascular system, liver, and gut. When you test your levels of estrogen, which can be done by blood, urine, or saliva, you can choose to replace the specific types of low estrogen (estradiol or estriol) or a combination of both.

The benefits of an optimal amount of estrogen are as plentiful as the downsides of insufficient estrogen. In the good column, estrogen is neuroprotective, heart protective, and bone protective. It has potent antioxidant properties, bolsters the metabolism, aids in the balance of circadian rhythms, increases mitochondrial biogenesis, reduces inflammation, and provides cellular protection. It also manages the glucose transport system which is crucial for insulin sensitivity. Another wonderful benefit of appropriate levels of estrogen is its facilitation of autophagy. I will delve into the world of autophagy in another chapter, but, for now, know that autophagy is essential for survival and optimal health. Estrogen levels begin to decline around the mid-thirties for most women, with some women maintaining their estrogen levels for longer. When this begins, a stage referred to as perimenopause begins and can last for years and be quite difficult for some women. On the list of negatives associated with diminished estrogen are mitochondrial dysfunction, neuroinflammation, synaptic decline, bone loss, insulin resistance, moodiness, weight gain, declining libido, and impaired sleep. While diminished estrogen can result in unpleasant symptoms, you don't want to become estrogen dominant either. Too much estrogen can cause a litany of issues and is often due to an inability to break down and excrete excess estrogen causing it to circulate in your body. Estrogen dominance can also be a result of insufficient progesterone levels, as those two hormones must be in balance.

There are many risks associated with estrogen dominance, and they include irregular ovulation, premature ovarian failure, polycystic ovary syndrome (PCOS), endometriosis, fibroids, vascular inflammation, neurologic inflammation, and estrogen toxicity. It is believed that there is a genetic component to how one metabolizes estrogen. To efficiently metabolize estrogen, you must have a healthy gut and a healthy liver. The process must include optimal breakdown of estrogen into its metabolites, and then the metabolites must be excreted out of the system through urine and stool. If this process isn't precise, the estrogen reenters the body in a reactive state and recirculates. Prolonged exposure to toxic estrogen metabolites can increase the risk of a poor health outcome. Metabolites are small molecules that are involved in metabolism.

The Environmental Working Group (EWG) site, which is a terrific resource, has identified the top twelve worst endocrine disruptors as being BPA, perchlorate, dioxin, atrazine, phthalates, lead, fire retardant, arsenic, glycol ethers, mercury, organophosphate pesticides, and PFCs, also known as perfluorinated chemicals.

If you decide to try bioidentical hormone replacement therapy, you should continue your own research and find a capable and knowledgeable practitioner.

If one is having difficulty balancing their hormones, they must investigate the cause and consider fixing the liver and the gut. Another source of hormonal imbalance is something called "endocrine disruptors." These are ubiquitous in our lives and are chemicals found in the air, water supply, soil, food supply, personal products, and manufactured products. They can't be metabolized like natural hormones and interfere with the critical hormonal balance.

Never take any kind of estrogen replacement orally. There are several modes of replacement, but oral estrogen should never be one. Estrogen taken orally is metabolized in the liver and can increase the risk of clotting, stroke, and some cancers. The other options are a patch applied directly onto your skin and changed biweekly, cream, gel, vaginal rings, suppositories, and pellets which are time released and require insertion subcutaneously. I have several girlfriends who swear that these pellets changed their lives, and they love the longer-lasting effects of this mode of hormonal replacement. One thing to consider with pellets is that you can't adjust the dose if it's incorrect as the pellets are inserted beneath your skin and can take several months to be fully absorbed. Something to consider with the cream replacement method is location. Many practitioners suggest applying the cream on your inner thigh but there are many other alternative locations and each spot impacts absorption differently. It has been suggested that cream applications can saturate the hormone receptors, resulting in a suboptimal outcome and it is preferable to place the cream on the vaginal mucosa. This belief varies greatly among practitioners, so it will be up to you to find the method for you.

Each one of the methods has pros and cons and the best approach is to determine which works best for your physiology. I do believe that if you decide to try HRT, you should use the bioidentical form as opposed to the synthetic form and the most critical aspect of HRT is finding the appropriate dose for you as an individual.

PROGESTERONE

If you are a woman and if you still have a uterus, you do not want to replace declining estrogen without balancing it with progesterone. Replacing estrogen alone when one has a uterus can increase the endometrial lining of the uterus and can contribute to a higher risk of cancer. Before I begin the discussion of progesterone, I need to briefly describe the sequence of hormone production. It begins with cholesterol, which I will explain further later. Cholesterol turns into pregnenolone and DHEA. Pregnenolone is known as the mother of all hormones and while it is a metabolite, it is a precursor in the synthesis of other hormones. Pregnenolone then produces progesterone. DHEA produces testosterone, estrone, and estradiol. Progesterone, in turn, produces cortisol and aldosterone. While a small amount of progesterone is made in your adrenal glands where it is turned into cortisol, most of it is released in your ovaries when a follicle containing an egg bursts open during ovulation. In males, progesterone is produced in the adrenal glands at much lower levels than in women and is involved in sperm development. Progesterone is the hormone that supports pregnancy, hence the similarity of its name to "pro-gestation." Its function is to prepare the uterus for the fertilized egg and to create peace and calm. It is secreted mainly in the second half of the menstrual cycle. The benefits of appropriate levels of progesterone are the regulation of mood, cognition, neurogenesis, collagen production and inflammation, maintenance of skin elasticity, reduction of PMS, bloating, and anxiety. It is also protective of the heart, brain, and bones, has anticancer properties, and can help you sleep better.

Low or suboptimal levels of progesterone can cause painful breasts, anxiety, depression, aggression, irritability, bloating, and headaches or migraines. Like estrogen replacement, progesterone replacement has been demonized extensively. Several studies have suggested that despite this demonization, progesterone may improve breast cancer survival rates.[115] There are also studies showing the potential reduction in colon cancer risk when replacing declining hormones.[116] The causes of declining progesterone are lifestyle factors such as diet, stress, excessive exercise, and menopause.

Along with the above-mentioned symptoms of low progesterone, one can become estrogen dominant as their progesterone declines and they can experience unpleasant symptoms. Unlike estrogen replacement, oral progesterone is a viable option. There is also the option of cream progesterone. Once again, it is preferable to use a natural form of micronized progesterone as opposed to the synthetic version.

TESTOSTERONE

Testosterone is an androgen, and both men and women produce it endogenously (produced by your body) at dramatically different levels. Men produce about forty times more testosterone than women do. Testosterone is produced in men in the testes and adrenal glands and in women in the ovaries and adrenal glands. Once testosterone is produced by the testes or the ovaries and adrenal glands, it enters the bloodstream as "free T," which is the bioavailable form that your body can use. If your blood tests reveal that you have high levels of total T, it doesn't mean that you also have high levels of bioavailable T. Ideally, you want about 2 percent of your total testosterone to be free. When too much free T converts into estradiol and DHT, your levels of bioavailable T decline and you are at a higher risk for health issues. Testosterone converts into estrogen through an enzyme found in multiple tissues in the body called aromatase. This process, aromatization, is your body's way of maintaining homeostasis and occurs primarily in men but also in women when their levels of testosterone become out of balance. While this process has also been found to control the amounts of cortisol the body uses to regulate the immune system, aromatase is a detrimental enzyme that you do not want in excessive amounts.

By menopause, testosterone levels in women have declined by about 50 percent. Over the last few decades in the US, there has been a substantial decline in testosterone levels in men. Recent clinical studies have not been able to pinpoint the precise reasons for this decline, but it is thought that they cannot be explained exclusively by health and lifestyle factors like smoking and obesity. One study suggests that there may be environmental factors to blame.[117] As we age, we become more inflamed due to, among other variables, an increase in inflammatory cytokines such as interleukin-6 (IL-6), tumor necrosis factor-alpha (TNF-alpha), and interleukin-1beta (IL-1β). These inflammatory cytokines decrease testosterone levels, but studies have found that testosterone replacement reduces these inflammatory markers in men.[118] There have also been clinical studies showing the benefits of testosterone replacement on the inflammatory markers of women. Men and women react quite differently to causes of inflammation.

The process of inflammation is slightly different in men and women in that an enzyme called phospholipase D causes increased inflammation as the enzyme increases. The immune cells of women produce nearly double the amount of pro-inflammatory substances than the immune cells of men. This enzyme, phospholipase D, is far less active in men than in women. Testosterone seems to suppress phospholipase D activity, and testosterone replacement diminishes this enzyme in female immune cells.[119]

Most studies on women and testosterone have been limited to the low sexual desire in women and one of these studies conducted in 2019 concluded that "there are insufficient data to support the use of testosterone for the treatment [for women] of any other symptom or clinical condition [other than HSDD (hypoactive sexual desire disorder)], or for disease prevention."[120] I found this conclusion both startling and conflicting based upon all of the anecdotal evidence for the support of testosterone replacement in women I have heard. I searched further and found studies concluding that, in fact, there is evidence that testosterone replacement can be efficacious for the treatment of endometriosis[121] and another study suggesting that testosterone use can be beneficial for pain associated with fibromyalgia.[122] Preexisting testosterone deficiency due to either environmental stress or genetic predisposition may explain why some individuals are more susceptible to chronic pain than others. I will concede that there is insufficient evidence to support the use of testosterone to enhance cognition but just because studies have not been conducted or haven't yet yielded positive results doesn't necessarily mean that it isn't worth pursuing further.

The benefits of sufficient levels and balanced testosterone in both men and women are plentiful. These benefits include the promotion of muscle mass, energy, endurance, libido, the protection of bones, the brain, heart, arteries, joints, skin, and immune function, and the reduction of stress, anxiety, depression, and oxidative stress. When testosterone levels are too high, too low, or simply unbalanced, insulin resistance can occur as well as fatigue, anxiety, depression, impaired sleep, poor memory, weak muscles, erectile dysfunction, and increased heart disease.

ALWAYS MONITOR THE DOSE OF BHRT

> If one wants to experiment with exogenous replacement of any hormones, they should seek out an experienced practitioner and aim to use the lowest physiological dose that yields the best results.

Supplements like acetylcarnitine, arginine, leucine, and glutamine and activities like weight lifting and even intermittent fasting have been shown to increase one's endogenous production of testosterone.

Consistent blood work should be performed to monitor and adjust the dose, as necessary. I believe that one should determine the function of their liver, kidneys, and overall health as well as identify their ultimate goals of replacement therapy before beginning. Bioidentical hormones in the form of estrogen, progesterone, and testosterone are all approved by the FDA. Since the bioidentical form has the same molecular structure as those produced endogenously, they do not have the same side effects as the synthetic hormones if appropriate doses are used. One should not use oral testosterone, and women need to be aware of the potential side effects of acne and increased body and facial hair. Adjusting the dose if these side effects occur usually resolves the issue. While no serious adverse effects have been noted, the safety of long-term use of hormone replacement has not yet been established.

ALCOHOL CAN LOWER TESTOSTERONE

One particularly interesting aside that I learned through my research is that alcohol can lower testosterone. In particular, the hops in beer are so estrogenic that they contribute to the decline of testosterone levels.

TEST YOUR HORMONES REGULARLY

Regarding testing, there are several options. You can test your hormones through blood, saliva, and urine. I believe strongly in the saying that you can't manage what you can't measure, so ideally you should do several types of testing. While blood tests are standard and often yield good and useful data, there is also the perspective that a blood test is merely a snapshot in time at the moment the blood was drawn and can vary according to what you ate, drank, how you slept, and how stressed you were immediately before the blood draw. Then there is the issue of the ranges. I suggest that you do not want to be in the "normal" range. Who is normal? The goal should be that which is optimal for you. You will have to pay close attention to your symptoms and how you feel. The gold standard in hormone testing that many doctors have yet to discover is called the DUTCH Test. It is an acronym that stands for "Dried Urine Test for Comprehensive Hormones." It looks at your hormone levels and how your body processes and metabolizes hormones. It gives far more useful information than blood or saliva tests. The hormones tested by this method are cortisol, cortisone, estradiol, estrone, estriol, progesterone, testosterone, DHEA, and melatonin. This test is not inexpensive, requires an experienced practitioner to decipher the results, and is not covered by insurance but reveals important information about you and your hormones. It is critical to know not only your hormone levels but also how your body is metabolizing your hormones. If your body is converting your hormones into damaging byproducts, you want to know this. Above all, you want to be your own health advocate. It is simply imprudent to delegate the entire process of your health care to a doctor. Get involved.

JANE'S STORY

Jane started to experience serious fatigue and brain fog beginning in her forties. Much to her dismay, she woke up tired, was groggy throughout most of the day, and fell into bed utterly exhausted. She never had any energy. She consulted doctor after doctor and was ultimately diagnosed with hypothyroidism and perimenopause. The doctors prescribed both thyroid medication and bioidentical hormone replacement. After taking the medications and hormones for a couple of months, Jane felt only slightly better. The doctors' solution was to increase the dosages of the medications and the hormones. This began a cycle of frustration.

Jane began her hormone odyssey by using an estradiol patch which required changing twice a week. Along with the patch, she was taking progesterone pills and testosterone cream. Determined to remedy this annoying issue, Jane decided to do frequent blood work to track the progress or lack thereof. When the blood work indicated only slight improvements in her hormone metrics, she experimented with different types of hormone replacement. Her next foray was into the area of pellets. The smallest dose of pellets containing estrogen and testosterone resulted in an unpleasant reaction which Jane was forced to endure for months until they were fully absorbed. Her next approach was the application of all three hormones in cream form. The prescribing doctor started her on the lowest dose, which was a twice-daily application of the three creams. This doctor had extensive experience in hormone replacement and was an ardent supporter of BHRT. In my opinion, despite her vast experience, the four different dosage levels were still not sufficiently personalized. Jane started on the lowest dose, twice a day, and tested her blood every three months for a year. She was concerned that her hormone numbers were quite high and didn't share her doctor's feeling that this was a great outcome. Several other doctors that Jane spoke with all felt that her numbers were too high.

She had no choice but to take matters into her own hands and began a course of self-experimentation. Her first action was to abandon the cyclical dose prescribed and try a static dose. A cyclical dose varies throughout the days of the month. In other words, each day calls for a different amount of hormone cream. The theory behind this protocol is that prior to the decline of our endogenous hormones, our bodies release different amounts each day and even at different times throughout the day. While this can't be duplicated precisely, it is thought that a cyclical dose comes close to mimicking our natural, youthful hormone production. A static dose is the same amount every day.

Jane found that the static dose didn't work for her as she began to experience hot flashes and sleep disturbances. She realized that returning to the lowest cyclical dose resulted in extremely high blood markers, so she decided to try doing the cyclical dose once a day instead of twice a day. She also experimented with the location of the placement of the creams. She tried placing the cream on her inner thigh, on her inner arm, on the back of her knee, and on her vaginal mucosa to test absorption.

Currently, Jane is feeling better. Her bone-crushing fatigue, hot flashes, and sleep disturbances have all improved. She doesn't feel that she has achieved perfect hormonal balance, but perhaps improvement is the best that she can achieve. Some women have greater success than Jane has had with BHRT, but she is happy for her improvement. She credits her amelioration to her dedication and willingness to experiment.

METABOLIC HORMONES

CORTISOL

> The three main metabolic hormones are cortisol, insulin, and thyroid.

Cortisol is a corticosteroid that comes from cholesterol. The precise pathway of cortisol release begins in the hypothalamus in the brain. Your hypothalamus sends a message to your pituitary, which in turn alerts your adrenal glands to make cortisol. The next step in this process is in the mitochondria. Cortisol and other steroid hormones are produced and metabolized by your mitochondria. Cortisol is a stress mediator, and it turns on and off when necessary. While cortisol helps the body adapt to stress, problems arise when the stress is prolonged, and the response doesn't turn off. That is when dysregulation and all of its attendant ills occur. While its main function is to increase circulating glucose, cortisol has paradoxical aspects in that, at the right level, it enhances the immune system, but, at too high of a level, cortisol can depress the immune system. It can be anti-inflammatory at the right level and pro-inflammatory at too high of a level.

Our brains evolved to recognize the threat of being chased by a tiger and to trigger several chemical reactions to ensure our safety.

The problem is that the threat of a tiger is no longer relevant today, but the amygdala in our brain responds to other threats, both real and imagined, in the same way.

Perhaps it sounds familiar to you that when perceiving something frightening, your breathing changes, your blood pressure changes, your heart rate increases, your muscles tense, and you may begin to sweat. This is called the "fight or flight response" and when stimulated by the sympathetic nervous system, triggers epinephrine and cortisol into your system to deal with the threat. The blood flow shifts from the major organs and moves into your arms and legs to prepare you to fight or flee the nonexistent tiger. One problem with this response is that the amygdala (the fear center in the brain) regulates perception and often what we perceive to be a threat is not an actual threat. Temperature, food, stress, environment, sleep, blood sugar, infection, inflammation, pain, toxins, and obesity are all examples of stimuli that impact the release of cortisol.

Cortisol resistance had been referred to for some time as "adrenal fatigue," but that term recently has been invalidated. It was thought that the constant

Cortisol is one of four hormones essential to life. Occasional spikes of cortisol throughout the day are to be expected but excess cortisol release must be avoided. When too much cortisol is released into the bloodstream with frequency, a negative feed loop is triggered and sends a message to the brain to stop making so much cortisol. The chronic release causes the normal turn-off switch to stop working because of excess stimuli and then cortisol becomes catabolic. When cortisol becomes catabolic, the breakdown of muscle occurs, inflammation increases, and cortisol resistance results. This is the beginning of the path to accelerated aging and chronic disease.

release of cortisol tired out one's adrenal glands, but the prevailing theory is that the problems occur in the hypothalamus, the pituitary, and the adrenal glands concurrently, and the new term is HPA axis dysregulation. All of this is a great example of the fact that nothing in the body occurs in isolation. There are always what are called "down-stream effects." When one event occurs, it triggers other events.

An example of this is the impact of dysregulated cortisol on the thyroid. Both low and high levels of cortisol interrupt thyroid function. There is also a direct impact of cortisol on insulin. The two are considered antagonists.

As with so many other functions in our body, circadian rhythms are at play with cortisol. It is considered a diurnal hormone and ideally spikes in the morning and wanes throughout the day, gradually decreasing at night. The cortisol spike in the morning is called the cortisol awakening response and should occur within the first thirty to sixty minutes after getting out of bed in the morning.

INSULIN

Insulin is another hormone that we could not live without. It is made by the pancreas and its function is to control blood sugar levels. It is an anabolic hormone and promotes growth, healing, and repair.

While most people attribute insulin's function to storing excess sugar in fat cells, it performs quite a few useful other functions. It protects against heart disease. It strengthens muscles and bones, helps maintain thyroid function, immunity, digestive and cognitive function, protects against neuroinflammation, and assists in the maintenance of overall hormonal balance. The key to insulin performing all of these important functions is that, like most everything, it must be balanced. You do not want too much insulin, and you do not want too little insulin. Too little insulin can result in type 1 diabetes, which is when the pancreas fails to produce sufficient insulin. Too much insulin results in type 2 diabetes and is due to insulin resistance.

When you eat food, the food is broken down into glucose. The glucose is released into your bloodstream and then it travels into your cells where it either is used to produce energy or is stored for future use. As you can guess, the type of food that you eat influences insulin release. When you eat too much sugar or carbohydrates, too much insulin is released and is stored as glycogen. This results in damaged blood vessels, inflammation, and the failure of the cells to use the glucose for energy production. The cells become resistant and then the pancreas tries to compensate by releasing even more insulin, leading to more inflammation, more fat, and a litany of things you want to avoid. The best way to avert this process is to either avoid excess sugar and carbohydrate consumption or, at the very least, balance this consumption with exercise and movement. There is a limited amount of storage space in our muscles and the liver for glucose storage, but there is no limit as to how much glucose we can store in body fat. Insulin resistance leads to diabetes, heart disease, cancer, obesity, high blood pressure, PCOS, bone loss, muscle loss, arthritis, migraines, stroke, and Alzheimer's disease.

CONSIDER INVESTING IN A CONTINUOUS GLUCOSE MONITOR

It is worth the effort to avoid insulin resistance.

You should take time to determine what your unique response to the glycemic index of different foods is. This index measures the effect that a particular food has on your blood sugar. For example, carrots and bananas, two seemingly benign and healthy foods, are both considered to be "high glycemic" foods but can

We are all genetically and physiologically unique and respond differently to everything.

trigger vastly different responses in individuals. The glycemic index is not the same for everyone. Two different people can have quite different responses to the same food. The best way to learn about your response is through a continuous glucose monitor (CGM). This is a device created for diabetics but has great utility for everyone. In my opinion, everybody should have a CGM for at least two weeks to learn about their physiological responses to food. Your doctor will have to give you a prescription for this, but most doctors will likely agree to do so once they understand your goal. The device is attached to either your upper arm or stomach through a needle for a period of two weeks. You can download an app on your phone that corresponds with the device and reads your blood sugar whenever you wave your phone using the sensor in the CGM. This is extraordinarily useful data to have on your path to optimal health. You should also know what your fasting glucose and insulin numbers are, and these can be learned through a routine blood test.

THYROID

It is estimated that between twenty and sixty million Americans, the majority of which are women, have some sort of thyroid disease. I have read that anywhere from 5–23 percent of Americans have one of four types of this disorder and many go undiagnosed. The four different types are hypothyroidism, which is insufficient thyroid hormone production; hyperthyroidism, which is overactive thyroid hormone production; thyroiditis, which is inflammation of the thyroid gland; and Hashimoto's thyroiditis, which is an autoimmune condition where the body attacks and damages the thyroid. The thyroid is a small butterfly-shaped gland located in the front of your neck adjacent to

The thyroid is the master gland of the body, and its function is to control and maintain metabolism, regulate body temperature and weight, and regulate energy transfer and production.

your trachea. This gland secretes two thyroid hormones: T4 (thyroxine) and T3 (triiodothyronine). The pituitary gland has a role here as well as it influences the amount of thyroid hormone in your bloodstream and secretes a thyroid hormone called TSH, or thyroid-stimulating hormone.

When one has hypothyroidism, the thyroid activity is low and causes everything in the body to slow down. Body temperature declines, rendering one's hands and feet persistently cold. Circulation slows, bowels slow, weight loss slows and depression, anxiety, and fatigue increase. One's skin and hair become very dry, the outer third of the eyebrows disappear, and memory and concentration are adversely impacted.

One of the important functions of the thyroid is to maintain cell function and stimulate the mitochondria. When one has hypothyroidism, this is no longer effective, and as the mitochondria slow down, so does protein synthesis and hormone metabolism. When one has low thyroid issues, it is often due to the inability of T3 getting into the cells. One of the reasons that so many people have undiagnosed hypothyroidism is that the laboratory reference tests used in most blood tests are out of date. What is called "normal" by antiquated data is now considered problematic. Functional medical doctors seem to have grasped this and when one's TSH, for example, falls into the antiquated normal range but is high considering current findings, then treatment is considered. Also, when getting a blood test if thyroid issues are suspected, be sure to test TSH, reverse T3, free T3, free T4, and the antibodies anti-TPO and anti-Tg.

Hyperthyroidism is also called Graves's disease and is when the thyroid gland makes more thyroid hormones than are necessary. Symptoms of this include irritability, sleep issues, weight loss, irregular heartbeat, increased appetite, and sometimes a noticeable goiter or swelling of the thyroid gland.

Hashimoto's thyroiditis is an autoimmune condition named for the Japanese surgeon who identified it in 1912. It is an autoimmune condition where the immune cells mistakenly attack the gland instead of protecting it. The thyroid becomes inflamed and can no longer produce enough thyroid hormone for your body to function properly. While the best treatment is to attempt to balance the immune system, before any treatment for this or any disorder takes place, it is essential to determine the cause of the imbalance or dysfunction first.

If one treats symptoms without first identifying the cause of anything, the problem will not be eradicated, and it will return. The causes of Hashimoto's could be issues with the hypothalamus, the pituitary, the liver, the kidneys, nutrient deficiencies, or cellular disrepair. The causes of hypothyroidism could be high estrogen, inflammation, infections, toxin exposure, or poor gut health. If you just take a pill or any kind of treatment without knowing the root cause, your improvement will probably be transient. Improving one's diet is always a good place to start. Eliminating all processed foods will improve many aspects of your health. You may have certain food sensitivities that are hard to determine. The best way is to do an elimination diet, which I described in chapter 7.

Thyroid physiology is quite complex. The thyroid hormone affects nearly all cells in the body. Usually, thyroid dysfunction can be traced to excessive cell stress and the cell danger response. This is a concept written about by Robert Naviaux and referenced elsewhere in this book. Thyroid issues are rarely due to one factor but rather they are due to multiple factors. This explains why so many people taking prescribed thyroid medication don't feel better. When your cells are faced with excessive cellular stress, they adapt by reducing thyroid physiology. Dr. Eric Balcavage, an expert in thyroid physiology, states, "Far too many people are told they JUST have a thyroid problem, when in reality the adaptation of thyroid physiology is the body's attempt to address the real problem in the body." He feels that untreated, or mistreated, thyroid issues can result in insulin resistance, diabetes, obesity, elevated lipids, compromised detoxification, fatty liver, renal dysfunction, GI dysfunction, and more.

I could go on and on talking about hormones and have only highlighted a small number of the hormones secreted by the human body. Not only are they incredibly fascinating, but they are essential to every function in the body. Rarely are our hormones in perfect balance and, like everything else, they decline as we age. Stress, viruses, heavy metal exposure, poor sleep, poor nutrition, digestive issues, and other things can all contribute to hormonal imbalances and the resulting increase in inflammation and reduction in metabolism. While there are some risks associated with BHRT, there are also risks in every single decision we make each day. I do not want to ignore that for some people, the risks far outweigh the benefits, but, for others, the benefits are worth the risks. Only you can decide what will make you most comfortable. We can support our declining hormones with BHRT and thyroid medications along with proper sleep, movement, hydration, stress reduction, and nutrition.

ACTION STEPS

- ➢ First, consult a knowledgeable, experienced practitioner in hormone replacement.
- ➢ Take careful note of your symptoms.
- ➢ Get a hormone panel done.
- ➢ Do a DUTCH Test to understand your metabolites.
- ➢ Experiment with different types and doses of BHRT to determine the best course of action for you.
- ➢ Always continue testing and monitoring.

CHAPTER 11

COLD THERMOGENESIS:
Highly Unpleasant but Effective

THE USE OF COLD THERAPY dates back to 1600 BC and is referenced in the most ancient medical text, known as the Edwin Smith Papyrus.[123] For some reason, the use of this therapeutic fell out of favor for centuries and around the 1980s began to reemerge. Many clinical studies are confirming the recurring interest in and benefits of cold therapy.

> Thermogenesis is defined as the process of heat production, and cold thermogenesis is the process of heat production because of cold exposure.

DIFFERENT TYPES OF COLD THERAPY AND THE MANY BENEFITS

Cold exposure includes cold showers; cold plunges into rivers, oceans, lakes, and bathtubs; wearing ice-cold vests specifically designed for this purpose; sleeping on a Chilipad with cold circulating water while you sleep; sleeping in a cold room; and cryotherapy. The multitude of benefits derived from cold therapy include increased blood flow and nitric oxide to the brain, decreased inflammation, improved immune system, mood improvement, increased metabolic rate, improved insulin sensitivity, improved sleep, reduced muscle soreness, and faster recovery from exercise.

COGNITIVE BENEFITS

Dr. Rhonda Patrick, in her report "Cold Shocking the Body," describes the benefit of cold exposure on the brain by explaining that exposure to the cold stimulates cold shock proteins that can repair damaged synapses. She goes on to say that cold exposure stimulates a release of norepinephrine, which positively affects focus, attention, and mood. There is anecdotal evidence that this kind of therapy can prevent and treat depression, which is credible because a lack of norepinephrine contributes to depression. Cold exposure also decreases cortisol levels and increases serotonin.[124] Further evidence of this brain benefit is confirmed by the fact that cold exposure tricks the brain into a fight-or-flight response. This triggers sympathetic activity in our autonomic nervous system, which results in increased focus and alertness.[125]

IMMUNE SYSTEM BENEFITS

The previously mentioned increase in norepinephrine reduces inflammation, which is nearly always a good thing. I say nearly and not always because as I have described in chapter 3, occasional, acute inflammation is necessary for survival. The

One of the best benefits of cold exposure is the immune system boost that one receives when consistently practicing cold thermogenesis. The immune system is optimized because inflammation is decreased.

other mechanism of immune system optimization is the increase in glutathione that occurs after cold exposure. Glutathione is the master antioxidant and critical to good health. It reduces oxidative stress, detoxifies, and boosts one's immune system. In addition to these immune boosters, frequent cold exposure increases white blood cells as well as T cells, which guard against illness.[126]

BROWN FAT VS. WHITE FAT

> Homeostasis is defined as "the tendency toward a relatively stable equilibrium." Our bodies are in a constant state of adjustment in search of this balance or homeostasis.

When we are exposed to cold, our bodies produce heat to warm us up and maintain our homeostatic optimal temperature of approximately 98.6 degrees Fahrenheit or 37 degrees Celsius.

The way that the body produces heat to maintain our homeostatic temperature when exposed to cold is by shivering and by producing brown adipose tissue, also known as brown fat. Brown fat is different from the white fat that most of us have in abundance. White fat is inert and is known to store energy, while brown fat is not inert but rather metabolically active and expends energy. The more brown fat one has, the more calories they burn and the lower their overall body fat percentage is.[127]

When we are cold, our body automatically reacts by producing more energy to keep us warm. Shivering when cold is compared to sweating when hot as two methods of maintaining a steady body temperature. This process burns more calories and fat and stimulates our metabolism. Our metabolic rate increases because of the activation of brown fat. The main function of brown fat is thermogenesis and the regulation of the body's energy expenditure. It functions more like muscles than like white fat. We used to believe that brown fat decreased over the first few years after birth. We no longer think this is true as studies have revealed that brown fat can be activated beyond infancy. Lean people have more brown fat than obese people, and young people have more brown fat than older people.[128],[129],[130]

POTENTIAL LONGEVITY BENEFITS

There is even some suggestion that exposure to cold temperatures could increase longevity. Several studies on both rats and worms have resulted in observing life extension of about 10–20 percent. This is explained by the fact that cold exposure speeds up one's metabolism, reduces chemical reactions, and triggers a gene that slows the rate of aging.[131] It is known that cold exposure triggers "cold shock proteins." These are multifunctional RNA/DNA binding proteins that assist with cell regeneration and repair and have the potential to turn on longevity genes.

It is quite common for athletes to apply ice locally on an injury or get into an ice bath or a cold plunge after exercise. While the way injuries are treated is continually changing based on evolving data, it is known that cold exposure can reduce muscle soreness and speed up recovery. This works because the cold causes vasoconstriction which is a narrowing of the arteries and the blood vessels. When these are narrowed, blood flow to the muscles is reduced and inflammation is decreased thus allowing for healing. I am sure that most of us are familiar with the sensation of our fingers, toes, and nose becoming very cold as the process of vasoconstriction moves the blood flow from our extremities to our core to maintain body temperature. One thing that must be pointed out is that there have been studies that suggest that cold exposure after certain types of exercise, such as weight training or resistance exercise, may block muscle building and defeat the goal of building muscles.[132] This is an area where additional studies need to be completed.

SLEEP BENEFITS

Another terrific benefit of cold exposure is improved sleep. Your body's core temperature drops when you sleep and a cool room helps to both facilitate this and to regulate your body temperature. Our internal body temperature affects our circadian clocks.[133] The Sleep Foundation recommends that one turn their thermostat to between sixty to sixty-seven degrees (15.5–19 degrees Celsius) at night for optimal quality of sleep.

HORMESIS

The simplest explanation for the efficacy of cold exposure is "hormesis." Hormesis is a fascinating concept which states that exposure to transient stress creates adaptation, which results in increased resilience.

This concept guides my quest for optimal health, and I think it should guide yours as well. Examples of this are exercise, intermittent fasting, cold, heat, some phytochemicals, and even low doses of radiation. The key is in the dose. Small doses of something, which at a much higher dose would do harm, cause the body to adapt to maintain homeostasis. A few things to consider are that you do not want to overdo cold exposure and you do not want to immerse yourself quickly. Immersion must be done gradually to avoid cold-shock response, which can trigger both cardiac and respiratory issues. You should consult your doctor before trying any of this and, in the meanwhile, if you are so inclined, I recommend doing further research in this area. Wim Hof, whom I referred to in chapter 9, believes strongly in the benefits of cold exposure but he refines the term by calling it "controlled cold exposure."

THE STORY OF WIM HOF

While I have dabbled with cold exposure on my own, the story about Wim Hof is far more fascinating than my story. His story begins with the tragic mental illness and ultimate suicide of his wife. To recover from his overwhelming pain and suffering from the loss of his wife, Wim became singularly focused on achieving greater resilience from stress. He did so with both breathing and extreme cold exposure. On his path, Wim learned how his body responded to extreme cold. He walked barefoot outside in the winter, exercised in the snow while wearing no clothes or shoes, and frequently climbed into a tub filled only with ice. One of the twenty-six Guinness World Records that he achieved was for the longest period of time spent in one of these ice baths—one hour, fifty-three minutes, and two seconds!

Some of the extreme measures that Wim took included swimming under the top layer of a frozen lake in Finland, running a marathon in the snow while barefoot, attempting to climb Mount Everest while wearing only shorts and boots, and successfully climbing Mount Kilimanjaro while wearing the same outfit.

Combined with his own form of breathing exercises, Wim's exposure to extreme cold allowed him to activate and control bodily reactions that have become dormant because of today's sedentary and comfortable lifestyle. He found that his methods resulted in a significant improvement in his mood, immune system, and overall resilience. He recounts the frequently achieved state of deep relaxation that was induced by his extreme cold exposure and breathing technique. Wim Hof is an obsessive extremist and refers to himself as "The Iceman." I would not suggest that anyone needs to go to the lengths that he does to achieve some improvement in their resilience. I would suggest, however, that one starts slowly, avoid overdoing it, and take small steps on their path to building resilience and reducing stress. There is a possibility that, depending upon the context, cold exposure could create stress if one were already in a vulnerable state physically or mentally. This illustrates another concept that should guide your quest for optimal health: context. I suggest that you always consider the context, or conditions that you face, before trying anything new or setting expectations.

In addition to Wim Hof's story, there are many anecdotal stories of people experiencing great improvement from leg pain, back pain, arthritis, anxiety, eczema, and even hay fever after beginning a routine of cold thermogenesis.

While I personally would not attempt to run a marathon in the snow barefoot or do most of the things Wim does, I do believe that we are all too comfortable and unaware of the long-term consequences of avoiding physical challenges. There is value in challenging ourselves to some degree of discomfort to wake up our minds and bodies.

ACTION STEPS

➢ Begin slowly. Slow but consistent exposure will allow your body time to acclimate.

➢ If you feel as though you are on the verge of getting sick, avoid cold exposure as your body may be too vulnerable.

➢ Do not ever force. Build up your tolerance slowly and gradually.

➢ Turn on the cold water for thirty seconds at the end of your shower. Increase the amount of time if you are able.

➢ Never do an excessive amount of cold exposure. Too much can have adverse effects—unless you are Wim Hof!

CHAPTER 12

LIGHT OPTIMIZATION:
Who Knew?

THERE IS NO DENYING THE benefits of electricity and the light it produces. This innovation has enhanced all of our lives by increasing productivity, safety, and convenience. We are just beginning to understand the impact of light on the brain, and it's not always beneficial.

While there is a need for further research, there are currently quite a few studies that confirm the connection between exposure to artificial light and health issues. Years ago, humans went to sleep within a short period after the sun set and awakened with the rise of the sun. Both in ancient times and currently in nonurban areas, there is a distinct period of darkness after the sun sets at night. In many urban areas today, there is perpetual light. We have evolved to need darkness to effectively repair and restore our bodies. Light changes your biology in both good and bad ways. The focus of my research is on blue light and red light. There are several spectrums in between which have an impact as well, but violet, green, and yellow lights do not have as extreme an impact as blue and red light.

ARTIFICIAL LIGHT EXPOSURE AFTER DARK

The cells in our eyes pick up light signals and send messages to our body clocks which affect our circadian rhythms. Melanopsin is a protein or photoreceptor in our eyes that is activated by bright light and is responsible for the suppression of melatonin. Artificial light includes fluorescent light, LED (light-emitting diode), and incandescent light and is composed of visible light, ultraviolet light, and infrared radiation. While incandescent light has the least amount of blue light, the UV and blue light in LED and fluorescent light have a great deal of potential for harm. Light is measured by wavelengths called nanometers (nm), and blue light is in the range of 450–500 nm.

There is evidence to support that poorly timed exposure to blue light throws off our circadian rhythms, suppresses the excretion of our endogenous melatonin, increases the release of cortisol at the wrong time, and increases the risk of not only several eye-related diseases (dry eye, cataracts, glaucoma, and age-related macular degeneration) but also cardiovascular disorders, sleep disorders, endocrine disorders, gastrointestinal disorders, mood disorders, and even cancer.[134]

While blue light is not inherently bad, the timing of exposure to blue light makes all the difference. We need blue light exposure during the day. The sun is a source of healthy blue light, which we need in appropriate doses. The problems arise, and there are many, when we are exposed to blue light at night after sunset. The constant flow of blue light into our eyes at night from electronic devices with screens and certain light bulbs send incorrect messages to our brain and trick it into thinking that it is daytime when it is nighttime.

WHICH LIGHT BULB IS BEST?

There appears to be some distinction between exposure to blue light emanating from cell phones, tablets, and computer screens over that which emanates from light bulbs. A study performed by the French Agency for Food, Environmental and Occupational Health & Safety (ANSES) concludes that blue light causes "toxic stress" to the retina. The study states, "exposure to an intense and powerful [LED] light is 'photo-toxic' and can lead to irreversible loss of retinal cells and diminished sharpness of vision." The report distinguishes not only between LED lights and electronic screens (which may or may not be accurate) but also between short- and long-term exposure.[135] Short-term exposure is defined as days to weeks, and long-term exposure is defined as months to years. I am not sure that this is a useful distinction since years have passed since people have been using LED bulbs and having their heads buried in their phones or tablets.

There is a conflict when choosing the right light bulbs. Both compact fluorescent light bulbs (CFLs) and LED light bulbs are promoted to be energy saving and better for the environment. The conflict arises because both emit a harmful light bandwidth. The list of potential harm from these types of bulbs is long and includes suppressing the immune system, insomnia, eye strain, and mitochondrial damage among other things. Fluorescent bulbs contain a filament made from mercury, which the manufacturers claim is in a small amount, but it seems prudent to avoid mercury as it is a known neurotoxin and small amounts add up. LEDs are quite high in blue light, and they flicker which when exposed to for a prolonged time can lead to health issues ranging from headache and impaired vision to seizures.[136] The flicker is a result of the light pulsating for energy efficiency and while the eye cannot directly see the flicker, there is a potential for damage to the nervous system. To optimize one's health, it is recommended to buy halogen or incandescent bulbs. They are cheaper, give off a warmer light, and have fewer health concerns.

When purchasing light bulbs, you can look at the color rendering index (CRI) to measure the relationship of how light affects color. Ideally, you want a full red spectrum (R9). Even the Illuminating Engineering Society (IES) points out the dangers of certain wavelengths of light. "Optical radiation detected by the retina impacts an individual's behavior, psychology, and perception of the environment. The position of the IES is to promote and encourage a more complete understanding of human responses to optical radiation leading to improved designs for all lighted environments."[137]

While there is some dermatological evidence that blue light is used beneficially for certain skin conditions, since exposure to it raises cortisol, it can result in inflammation which can be potentially damaging to the skin. There is also evidence that blue light can accelerate aging and decrease collagen. I suggest that both context and dose should inform your decisions regarding blue light.

LIGHT SUPPRESSES MELATONIN

I found only one study presenting an opposing view about the harmful effects of blue light. This study was from the UK and was published in *Cell*.[138] I was not particularly impressed by the conclusions of the study on mice. For one thing, animal studies are not always the best evidence for that which happens in humans. While the study questions the validity of harm resulting from blue light, they conclude that yellow hues, instead of blue hues, have deleterious effects. A review of the study published in *Time* magazine on January 10, 2020, talks about the contradictory evidence but also states that "there is a valid scientific basis to the idea that blue light interrupts sleep, since research consistently shows that light of any kind suppresses melatonin and blue light may do so to an especially extreme degree." It is emphasized that the spectrum of light, brightness, and duration of exposure all matter and contribute to the degree of resulting harm.

MANAGE YOUR LIGHT EXPOSURE

One must manage their light exposure to achieve optimal health and performance. One way to easily reduce one's nighttime exposure to blue light is to get blue-light-blocking glasses. There are several commercially available brands in both prescription and nonprescription. Be aware that these glasses come in clear, yellow, and orange, and the different lenses block different amounts of blue light. Another way is to switch out one's light bulbs to incandescent and in your bedroom replace your nightstand bulb with a red bulb. This will imitate the wavelength of the sun setting and be more restorative for your eyes at night. There are apps to change your smartphone, tablet, and computer screens to red hues in the evening. There are also several apps that will measure lux to optimize your lighting. Lux tells you how much light falls on a certain area. It measures the degree of brightness detected by the human eye and can help avoid an environment that is too bright for your eyes. Overall, the goal is to block as much blue light after sunset as possible and to sleep in a very dark room.

RED LIGHT

While this area of science is known by several names, including red light therapy, infrared light therapy, low-level laser (light) therapy (LLLT), and photobiomodulation, it has not yet

> As harmful as blue light at night is, red light is known to be restorative and can repair damage.

achieved the wide acceptance that it should. I suspect that one day soon, it will be embraced because its benefits are numerous, there are no known side effects, and there are over five thousand clinical studies in support of its use. In many countries throughout the world, red lights have been used therapeutically for years. Interestingly, there are a lot of Russian studies on red light therapy's benefits, but most are not translated into English. This is not a new field of science, as evidenced by the Nobel Prize in Physiology or Medicine in 1903 awarded to Niels Ryberg Finsen for his use of light therapy to treat disease. In the last fifty years, both the use and study of photobiomodulation have increased. It is still not considered to be "mainstream," in part, because it doesn't require a prescription and is not very expensive. Conventional medicine is very tied to the pharmaceutical industry and both are profit motivated.[139]

MITOCHONDRIAL BENEFITS

The explanation for the vast benefits of this light therapy is that while all wavelengths of light stimulate mitochondria, red and infrared light penetrates the tissue most efficiently. Mitochondria are a critical component of health and are defined as organelles that are the power generators of the cell. They convert oxygen and nutrients into ATP (adenosine triphosphate) which provides energy and is essential to function and to survive. When you improve your mitochondrial health, the result is an overall improvement in the body's health and performance.

Red light is within 630–850 nm, which is low, and while it penetrates the dermis, one cannot feel it as it doesn't generate heat upon exposure. We can see the red wavelengths, but our eyes do not have the ability to see the near-infrared wavelengths. Different wavelengths affect the body at a cellular level. The synergistic effect of the two different wavelengths penetrates the tissues at different levels and produces the most optimum outcome.

Red and infrared light are known to increase both the number and the function of our mitochondria. The mechanism by which this is done is that as the mitochondria absorb the red and NIR light, they produce an enzyme called cytochrome c oxidase, which then induces the mitochondria to produce ATP for cellular use and decrease oxidative stress. The general result is cellular repair and healing.

NITRIC OXIDE AND CIRCULATION

One of the beneficial aspects of this treatment is the increase in one's circulation. In 1993, Duke University researchers discovered the connection between light therapy, vasodilation, and blood flow. In 1998, the Nobel Prize in Physiology or Medicine was awarded to Robert F. Furchgott, Louis J. Ignarro, and Ferid Murad "for their discoveries concerning nitric oxide as a signalling molecule in the cardiovascular system." Red blood cells carry a gas called nitric oxide and infrared light releases this gas from the red blood cells at the site of the light treatment. Nitric oxide dilates blood cells and improves blood flow. The light treatment increases vasodilation (blood flow) by increasing nitric oxide, and, in turn, the nitric oxide, in a circular fashion, increases blood flow. The role of nitric oxide is involved in three main pathways. They are endothelial, neuronal, and lymphatic.

THE FIELD OF PHOTOBIOMODULATION

A preeminent expert in the field of photobiomodulation is Michael Hamblin, PhD. He runs a photomedicine lab at Massachusetts General Hospital, is an Associate Professor of Dermatology at Harvard Medical School, and is a member of the Affiliated Faculty of Harvard-MIT Division of Health Sciences and Technology. As you can see, he is extraordinarily well credentialed, and his research focus is on photomedicine and its connection to disease. He has written and cowritten hundreds of peer-reviewed studies on the benefits of photobiomodulation. His papers reveal the results of studies on light therapy and the benefits for the brain, for the immune system, for skin, for chemotherapy side effects, diabetes, wound healing, and muscle recovery, to name just some of the benefits.

He has studied patients with traumatic brain injury, stroke, oxygen deprivation resulting from heart attacks, dementia, anxiety, PTSD, and depression. His conclusions are truly remarkable as he shows that the brain pathways can be remodeled after treatments, and while some of his trials are small, they have great outcomes and show the possibilities of improving outcomes without resorting to pharmaceuticals that can have long-term adverse effects. He explains that near-infrared light can penetrate through the skull and affect oxygen and blood flow into the brain.

Hamblin asserts strongly and with conviction that this type of noninvasive therapy can change the immune system from pro-inflammatory to anti-inflammatory, which is key to optimal health. This is accomplished by increasing blood flow and circulation to damaged tissues, reducing oxidative stress, and boosting ATP to facilitate cellular energy production. Tissues heal and regenerate faster and pain is eased. He also points out that photobiomodulation is a safe and effective alternative to NSAIDs or prescription anti-inflammatory drugs that can have side effects.

There is also a great deal of science supporting the benefits of light therapy on the skin, wound healing, sleep quality, and muscle performance. The skin antiaging benefit is due to the stimulation of collagen synthesis in the dermis by photobiomodulation. While this all seems almost too good to be true, it isn't. The light stimulates our cells to do what they were meant to do and triggers the signaling pathway which causes gene expression and potentially results in long-lasting beneficial changes.[140] While the optimal treatment frequency and duration will depend upon what you are attempting to optimize, one could safely have a daily ten-minute treatment and receive multiple benefits.

To illustrate the potential harm of artificial light, I want to share the story of one of my sons. My oldest son is a gamer. When he was a young boy, his best friend's dad introduced him to a series of video games that consumed a huge amount of his free time. The games that captured my son's interest are described as real-time strategy video games. The games were based on events beginning in the Stone Age in Europe, Asia, and Africa. I was horrified by this hobby but tried to learn about the industry. I tried to assuage my dismay by hoping that my son would learn about history and that the time he spent playing would be somewhat educational. It turns out that there are beneficial lessons from this seemingly time-wasting hobby. My son learned collaboration, as he was a part of a team, he learned strategy, persistence, critical thinking, and problem-solving. After observing his total and complete obsession with video games, I tried to persuade him to learn how to code and to create an educational video game. Well, that went exactly nowhere! He had no interest in coding and even less interest in creating an educational video game. You are probably wondering what this story has to do with a chapter about "light optimization." Most of my son's gaming took place after dark. As this chapter reveals, the excessive, and I cannot emphasize the word *excessive* enough, exposure to artificial light at night poses a great risk of harm. My son experienced terribly dysfunctional circadian rhythms. He developed a serious sleep disorder from staying up way too late in front of a computer. He had brain fog, headaches, and weight gain. While he is still not out of the woods in terms of his circadian rhythm dysfunction, he follows certain steps that have vastly improved his situation. First thing in the morning, or rather, his concept of "morning," he gets outdoor sun exposure. At night, he uses the red-screen function on his computer and cell phone, and he wears blue-light-blocking glasses. He is aware of the harms of artificial light exposure and is working to limit it.

ACTION STEPS

> ➢ Get early-morning sun exposure upon waking.

> ➢ Get blackout drapes for your bedroom.

> ➢ Wear blue-light-blocking glasses after dark.

> ➢ Turn on the red-screen function on your computers, devices, and smartphones.

> ➢ Switch your light bulbs.

CHAPTER 13

HYDRATION:
Essential for Optimal Functioning

ONE OF THE MAIN FUNCTIONS of water is to aid in the transmission and absorption of vitamins, minerals, and nutrients into the cells. Other functions are assisting in the proper digestion of food, detoxification, and the excretion of waste products. Our bodies produce a large amount of metabolic waste. It is critical for this waste to be excreted, and water facilitates this process through the mechanisms of sweat, urine, breath, and stool. When we are not hydrated, the metabolic waste doesn't get excreted efficiently and it builds up, which leads to a variety of adverse issues. These include muscle cramping, constipation, and blood vessel constriction, which in turn leads to the increase of blood pressure and impaired cognitive function. It cannot be overemphasized that hydration is a critical component of optimal health.

WATER CONTENT OF OUR BODY

Our bodies are primarily composed of water, and all biological systems depend on water. While the numbers differ somewhat, the rule of thumb is that the human body is between 55–75 percent water by mass. Our muscles are 75 percent water, our brains are 80 percent water, our lungs are 80 percent water, and our skin is 65 percent water. The molecules in our body are 99 percent water.[141] Giuseppe Vitiello, a professor in quantum field theory in Italy, explains that as the brain converts glucose from the blood into oxygen and energy, it produces water. A human brain contains about one liter of water and produces about fifty milliliters of water every twenty-four hours.

Our brains are extremely sensitive to water levels. A mere 2 percent of dehydration can reduce cognitive function and, in particular, performance in tasks that require attention, psychomotor, and immediate memory skills.[142]

As we age, the water content of our body decreases. Our blood and other bodily fluids are made up of water, and when we are dehydrated, these fluids become thicker, and the ability to absorb minerals and nutrients decreases. One of the reasons for muscle cramps is that dehydration alters the balance of electrolytes such as sodium, calcium, and potassium. Your body requires certain minerals to be able to absorb and use the water consumed. If you don't have these minerals and electrolytes, the cells can't absorb the water. Many of these important minerals are lost through sweat, urine, and other bodily functions.

DEHYDRATION CAN BE DEADLY

Water is essential for our survival as it supports and maintains every cellular biochemical function. These include muscle contractions, cell division, nerve conduction, and many others.[143] While one can survive for a long time without food, one will die after approximately three days without water. Despite the widely known fact that proper hydration is one of the many foundations of optimal health, 75 percent of Americans are chronically dehydrated. Dehydration is defined as the excessive loss of body water. It occurs when your body is losing more water than it is absorbing. There is a wide range of water loss, and if the amount exceeds 15 percent of one's total body water content, it can result in death. Chronic dehydration slows down the metabolism, increases fatigue, stimulates inflammation, increases cortisol levels, and increases the risk of certain diseases.[144]

> Water is essential for our survival as it supports and maintains every cellular biochemical function.

There is a fascinating book called *Your Body's Many Cries for Water* written by Dr. Fereydoon Batmanghelidj. While in jail for nearly three years, as a political prisoner, this Iranian doctor conducted extensive research on the dangerous effects of dehydration on one's health. He found that the efficiency of every single bodily function is dependent upon the intake of and absorption of water. His research revealed that dehydration causes asthma, allergies, arthritis, angina, premature aging, pain, hypertension, headaches, weight gain, and depression to name just a few!

FAT STORAGE INCREASES WHEN DEHYDRATED

When you are dehydrated, you store fat. The explanation for this is revealed through a look at the various functions of our organs. Your kidneys are supposed to filter your blood. Your liver is supposed to metabolize your stored fat. When you are dehydrated, your kidneys can't do their job efficiently, so your liver has to pitch in to help with the blood filtering. When the liver has to step in to help out with the job of the kidneys, it can no longer efficiently do its job of metabolizing fat. Both your endocrine system and its production of the fat-burning hormone, HGH (human growth hormone), as well as your production of lipase, the enzyme necessary for fat metabolism, become impaired by dehydration. The converse of this is true. There is a connection between increased hydration and weight loss. A study by Simon N. Thornton published in the *Frontiers in Nutrition* journal suggests that the weight loss from increased hydration is a result of eating less food and increased lipolysis (fat loss). The mechanism responsible for this is an increased metabolism leading to increased mitochondrial function.

There was a study conducted in the UK that found that dehydration is the number one cause of fatigue and can interfere with one's ability to focus and think clearly. The study found that driving while dehydrated can be as dangerous as driving while drunk.

ADDITIONAL RESULTS OF DEHYDRATION

There is increasing evidence that even mild dehydration may play a role in various morbidities.[145] When we are dehydrated, our bodies react by increasing histamine production, and this can contribute to both asthma and allergies.[146]

SYMPTOMS OF DEHYDRATION

The symptoms of dehydration vary according to the severity of water loss. They begin with thirst, headache, and fatigue. As water loss continues, constipation, dry mouth, dizziness, and infrequent urination become apparent. When the water loss becomes greater, the symptoms include dry skin, muscle cramps, sunken eyes, dry mucous membranes, confusion, seizures, and potentially death.

You do not want to wait until you are thirsty because the sensation of thirst is the first sign of dehydration. While dehydration is often overlooked as a cause of discomfort or disease, it's an easily remedied condition and improvements occur quickly. It takes approximately forty-five minutes to rehydrate. If you drink water on an empty stomach, it can enter your bloodstream in around five minutes. If you drink water while eating, digestion of food occurs first and prolongs the absorption of water by about forty-five minutes on average.[147,148] Ayurvedic principles have promoted drinking water thirty minutes before eating to avoid interfering with digestion and to absorb the water efficiently.

HOW MUCH WATER SHOULD YOU BE DRINKING?

For years we have all heard that we need to drink eight glasses of water every day. It turns out that this is just an average because the goal is to replace the amount of water that we lose throughout the day. There are so many factors that must be taken into consideration as to the appropriate quantity of water one must drink daily. Consider what climate you live in, how active you are, your age, your size, how much you sweat, and how frequently you urinate to determine your optimal quantity of water intake. While many experts state that coffee and tea should not contribute to your total volume of fluid intake because they are dehydrating in and of themselves, it turns out that may not be accurate. The Center for Disease Control includes coffee, tea, and water-rich fruits and vegetables as part of one's daily fluid intake. Foods like celery, melon, cucumber, and lettuce have a high water content and contribute to your overall water intake. An easy way to monitor your fluid balance is to check your urine output. The darker the color of your urine, the more dehydrated you are, and the optimal color should be that of light straw.

WATER QUALITY

Just like food, the quality of your drinking water matters. While there are several different types of water, tap water is not the best choice for drinking. In most areas, tap water is filled with environmental toxins and chemicals. There is insufficient regulation and oversight of municipal water. Analysis of tap water in many areas has revealed the presence of chlorine, fluoride, bromide, prescription drugs, herbicides, flame retardants, microplastics, and even radioactive chemicals from the 2011 Fukushima nuclear accident. There have been studies highlighting the connection between elevated fluoride concentrations in drinking water and neurotoxicity, particularly in children.[149] The countervailing argument tends to be from the dental industry, the claim of which is that fluoride is necessary to prevent tooth decay. This argument is not as compelling as it once was as science advances, and we learn other nontoxic methods of oral hygiene. The WHO has declared that there is no difference in cavities among people in countries with fluoridated water and those in countries without fluoridated water. Whatever you choose to believe, common sense dictates that as your exposure to toxic chemicals in your water increases, so will your health issues.

TYPES OF WATER

Different types of water to consider are ozonated, ionized (or alkaline), and hydrogen enriched. Despite its fad-like embrace, I won't spend any time on alkaline water other than to say it is ineffective. You can't alter the pH of your blood by drinking alkaline water. Your body regulates its blood pH in a very narrow range because all of our enzymes are designed to work at pH 7.4. If your pH varied a great deal, you would die. The pH of your urine is a slightly different story. Urine tends to be acidic, with a pH of 6, and what you eat and what you drink does have the potential to alter the pH of your urine. Additionally, alkaline water is not good for your gut microbiome because lactic acid and butyric acid control the growth of pathogens by lowering the pH of the intestines. This is an example of widespread misinformation that at best could do nothing positive but at worst may contribute some harm. Speaking of the acid/alkaline balance, it is good to know that sparkling water is ten times more acidic than flat water and may be harmful to your tooth enamel. Recently, it has been revealed that several popular brands of sparkling water contain levels of PFAS that exceed safety standards. PFAS, also known as per- and polyfluoroalkyl substances are human-made chemicals that are referred to as "forever chemicals" due to their inability to break down in the body or the environment. Consumer Reports, a nonprofit watchdog organization, did a full report on this issue.[150] It is important to note that the dose makes the poison. In other words, occasionally drinking sparkling water will not result in immediate harm. It's the consistent and multiple exposures to toxic chemicals that add up and result in harm.

OZONATED WATER

Ozonated water is quite controversial. It is not supported by the FDA or by big pharmaceutical companies in the US but people in other countries have been drinking it for years. The controversy ranges from it having tremendous healing and therapeutic benefits to being ineffective or harmful. It is accepted that breathing ozone can be harmful, so don't confuse that with drinking ozonated water. Ozone is a unique combination of gas and water which is referred to as an unstable form of oxygen. It has three atoms of oxygen which are bonded together, O_3, unlike the oxygen we breathe, which has two atoms of oxygen, or O_2. Because of its instability, ozone water acts as an oxidant in the body making it a free radical which can lead to cellular damage. The reality is that we need a balance of both oxidants and antioxidants. Oxidants help destroy pathogens in our body and are essential if they don't exist in abundance. Some believe that drinking ozonated water kills bacteria, viruses, and fungi; breaks down synthetic chemicals; provides more oxygen to the brain; improves the immune system; reduces inflammation; and can have anticancer properties. While there are quite a few clinical studies on ozonated water, there are even more anecdotal reports on its benefits.

HYDROGEN-ENRICHED WATER

Hydrogen-enriched water is water with extra hydrogen molecules added to it. Hydrogen is a flammable, colorless, odorless, nontoxic gas. It is worth pointing out that hydrogen (H) is in the first position on the periodic table of elements. Molecular hydrogen is three times denser than gasoline and is a great alternative energy source. This form of water is believed to have promising preventive and therapeutic effects for the treatment of a variety of diseases. Despite not yet being widely adopted as a treatment, this is not pseudoscience. There are over three hundred peer-reviewed studies on the benefits of hydrogen-enriched water. It is thought that the benefit of this water is due to its ability to penetrate the cell and mitochondria more efficiently than any other antioxidant. The explanation for this is that hydrogen is the smallest molecule that there is, is a neutral molecule, and also is devoid of any polarity. For those reasons, it has high cellular bioavailability which is essential for cell membrane penetration. Water alone is neutral but has polarity so it cannot go through the cell membrane by itself. It must use "aquaporins," which are water channels, or membrane proteins that help transport water between cells. Only a small number of substances can penetrate the inner mitochondrial membrane, and molecular hydrogen is one of those substances. Mitochondria represent one of the most, if not the most, important, life-sustaining components of our biology.

The areas that molecular hydrogen impacts are inflammation and oxidation. Both are explained in detail in another chapter, but, as a reminder, you don't want too much or too little of either inflammation or oxidation. The goal is neither to suppress nor to increase either of those but rather to modulate or balance both. This is where the brilliance of molecular hydrogen comes in. It can either increase or decrease inflammation and oxidation as needed. We see again and again that achieving a homeostatic balance of everything, including inflammation, oxidation, and even hydration is key.

Molecular hydrogen has a high safety profile, unlike many other frequently recommended supplements. It aids in cell signaling, metabolism, and gene expression and triggers an increase in our body's own antioxidant system. Its reported benefits include a decrease in inflammation, a decrease in oxidative stress, weight loss, improved athletic performance, improved oral health, wound healing, improved skin health, improved kidney function, and improvement in several diseases such as rheumatoid arthritis, type 2 diabetes, and depression. One of the many interesting clinical studies to review is called "Hydrogen-rich water for improvements of mood, anxiety, and autonomic nerve function in daily life" by Kei Mizuno and associates, published in the journal *Medical Gas Research.*

One can consume this type of water by pouches, bottles, pills placed in water, or by a hydrogen water machine. Regarding the appropriate dosage, it is suggested that one take a clinically relevant dose from a trusted manufacturer. My approach to dosage is always to begin with a small dose and gradually increase, taking note of any adverse side effects. If you are so inclined to learn more about this, I recommend going to the Molecular Hydrogen Institute website and learning from the scientists.

WATER FILTRATION SYSTEMS

As I previously mentioned, one must filter their tap water to eliminate toxic chemicals and pesticides. While Berkey filters, reverse osmosis systems, and even distilled water remove many toxins and impurities, they are not effective at eliminating pesticide residues, which are a big problem for our gut microbiome. The other issue with these filters is that they remove minerals along with the toxins. This can be remedied by adding back trace minerals or using electrolyte powder. Electrolytes include sodium, potassium, magnesium, and calcium, and they are important to consume because they help transport waste to be excreted. Drinking coconut water is a great way to ingest potassium, vitamins, minerals, and electrolytes. It must be noted that while a whole-house filtration system is expensive, it is most effective at removing what needs to be removed. The Berkey filter, other commercial filters, and bottled water in plastic water bottles are unable to filter out fluoride, and bottled water has the added negative factor of containing BPA or BPS and BPF, all of which have proven to be harmful. On the topic of bottled water, nearly all brands are contaminated with microplastics including polypropylene, nylon, and others.

> There has even been a study that showed that plastic particles were found in over 80 percent of global tap water as well as in many brands of beer and even in sea salt.

One can add a pinch of Himalayan salt to their drinking water, which will help your cells absorb the water better.

MY STORY

When I was younger, I would get debilitating migraine headaches. The only advice I was given was to avoid eating dark chocolate, cured meats, hot dogs, drinking red wine, and all other food and drinks containing nitrates. I followed the advice and continued to get migraines. I was fortunate in that my migraines only occurred about half a dozen times a year, unlike some people who suffer far more frequently.

One of my most memorable migraines happened when I was on a five-day bicycle trip. I was loving every minute of the trip until day three. I had been so riveted by the beautiful scenery, camaraderie, and the exhilaration of the exercise that I completely neglected my hydration. Somehow, I managed to endure with extraordinarily little water intake for the first three days and then my neglect caught up to me with a vengeance! By the end of day three, my head was pounding so hard that I had to miss dinner and retreat to my hotel room in complete darkness. Thankfully, a good night's sleep and some water helped, and I was ready to continue the next day. I realized how terribly dehydrated I was and began drinking water more consistently, not just for the rest of the trip, I had made my water consumption a priority from there forward. I am happy to report that I rarely get headaches anymore.

A word of caution: be careful not to overdo your water consumption. If you drink too much water in a short time, there is the potential for diluting your blood stream's sodium content and leading to hyponatremia, which you want to avoid. When you drink water, do so slowly as opposed to guzzling. Slow water consumption gives your cells time to absorb the water. There are even several smartphone apps to help you remember to constantly drink water throughout the day. Some of these apps are Daily Water Tracker Reminder; Hydro Coach; WaterMinder; Water Drink Reminder; iHydrate; AQUALERT: Water Tracker Daily, and Plant Nanny.

ACTION STEPS

➤ Drink water immediately upon waking.

➤ Continue drinking water throughout the day. Small amounts, frequently.

➤ Filter your water.

➤ Add minerals and electrolytes to your water.

➤ Beware of drinking too much water; hyponatremia, a severe dilution of sodium levels, can occur.

➤ Eliminate sugary drinks.

➤ Track your water consumption using one of several available apps.

CHAPTER 14

FASTING:
Reset Your System

FASTING FOR DIFFERENT DURATIONS HAS been utilized for millennia by many cultures. Historically, the motivation for fasting was primarily religious and spiritual, but, somewhat recently, the health and longevity benefits of fasting have been studied.

Most of the studies focus on the links between nutrition and genes that regulate cellular protection and regeneration. It is now accepted that fasting is an effective tool for healing.

Some of the exciting findings from the clinical studies have found that fasting triggers changes in metabolism and gene expression, reduces the risk of chronic disease, and has the potential to extend lifespan.

DIFFERENT TYPES OF FASTING

Fasting is an umbrella term that describes a multitude of different adjustments one can make to their feeding schedules or different types of food restrictions. Caloric restriction is just as it sounds and is defined as reducing the number of calories you ingest. Intermittent fasting has a few descriptions and can mean alternate-day fasting as well as compressed feeding windows or timed eating. Time-restricted eating describes the fasting method of compressing your feeding window into specific hours, like twelve-twelve or sixteen-eight hours. In other words, eat during a twelve-hour window and fast for twelve hours, or eat only within an eight-hour window and fast for sixteen hours. This is my favorite type of fasting and is not difficult to accomplish. The limitation is not on the amount or type of food that you eat but rather on the hours in the day spent eating. If you think about it, the word "breakfast" means the meal that breaks your fast. It is embedded in the word, and it implies that you have stopped eating for a period. Unless you have severe hypoglycemia, hormone imbalance, thyroid issues, or some other condition, the advice that we used to receive about maintaining our blood sugar by eating small meals every two hours turns out to be completely the opposite of what studies find.

> Every time we eat and digest food, we are requiring our biology to work hard. If there are no extended breaks in the digestive process, the body doesn't have the chance to rest and repair, not to mention the suppression of the release of human growth hormone resulting from frequent eating and overeating. Studies show that fluctuations between eating and fasting are required for optimal metabolic function.

Other modes of fasting are alternate-day fasting, twenty-four-, thirty-six-, forty-eight-, or seventy-two-hour fasts, or even longer. There is also what is called the 5:2 diet, which is described as eating how you normally do and either going without food or just having one meal a day for the other two days of the week. A favorite type of fasting of mine is the "fasting-mimicking diet" created by a longevity expert named Dr. Valter Longo. There is also a religious-inspired fast, exemplified by Muslims during Ramadan. This involves no eating or drinking during the day and feasting at one meal at night for thirty days. When one is amid the fasting period only water, black coffee, and tea will not interfere with the beneficial biological process resulting from fasting. There are several "juice fasts," but the results are not the same as interrupting the digestive process altogether. One should consult their doctor before embarking on any kind of a fast and children under eighteen years old, the elderly, pregnant and nursing mothers, and those with certain preexisting conditions should refrain from fasting.

BENEFITS OF FASTING

Decades of clinical studies have found that there are numerous benefits of fasting. Some of the health conditions that have been found to improve from fasting are obesity, type 2 diabetes, cardiovascular disease, cancers, and neurological disorders. In addition to weight loss, improved gut flora, and improved blood lipid and glucose control, fasting benefits overall metabolic health.

When you eat, insulin levels rise, excess glucose is stored in the liver as glycogen, and what can't be stored in the liver is stored as fat. The exact opposite process occurs when you fast. Fasting causes insulin levels to drop, and your body burns stored energy. First, glycogen, a form of glucose, stored in the liver, is burned, and then fat is burned. The key becomes switching from burning glucose to burning fat, which we know is the body's stored food energy.

THE IMPACT ON GLUCOSE WHEN YOU EAT AND WHEN YOU FAST

Since our sedentary habits have increased along with our food consumption, it can safely be said that most of us eat more than we need for energy use.

KETONES

The mechanism by which this occurs is through the production of ketones. Ketones are an alternative energy source, known as energy substrates, which are made in the liver from stored fats. These are effective energy sources for the brain, muscles, and other tissues and organs with high metabolic rates. Not only do ketones improve metabolism, but they have also been shown to increase longevity. While the body produces ketones during fasting, that is not the only way to increase their production. The alternative way to stimulate ketone production is the currently popular "ketogenic diet." So many people love this diet because they quickly lose a lot of weight and claim to feel great. The problem with this diet is that it requires exceedingly high quantities of fat intake which, depending upon your genetics, could be quite harmful. While it is recommended that if one tries this diet, they should only remain on it for no longer than six weeks or cycle in and out of it, many have adopted it as a lifestyle without regard to the long-term implications. It is believed that when one is in ketosis, the metabolic state describing the release of ketone bodies, there is an associated reduction in risk of metabolic disease, diabetes, and cardiovascular disease.

EIGHTEEN HOURS TO KETONE ENERGY

A study conducted in 2019 confirmed the benefits of intermittent fasting and stated that evidence is accumulating that eating within a six-hour period and fasting for eighteen hours can trigger a metabolic switch from glucose-based to ketone-based energy, with increased stress resistance, increased longevity, and a decreased incidence of diseases, including cancer and obesity.[151]

HUMAN GROWTH HORMONE

Another hormone that is affected by fasting is human growth hormone (HGH). This hormone stimulates metabolism and cell repair, increases muscle growth and strength, increases bone density, decreases fat, and can help us recover from injury and disease. This is a hormone that we make endogenously until we begin aging and choosing less-than-stellar lifestyle habits. When we eat frequently throughout the day and when we overeat, we suppress the release of HGH. Fasting, on the other hand, causes our insulin levels to decrease, our metabolism to speed up, and our production of HGH to increase. There are other ways to increase the very antiaging HGH but most include taking different supplements. Improving your sleep, doing HIIT (high-intensity interval training) exercise, and intermittent fasting are all ways to accomplish this improvement without side effects.

NEUROPROTECTIVE BENEFITS OF FASTING

Even a brief period of food restriction can induce widespread upregulation of autophagy, which is believed to be neuroprotective. The nutrient sensing involved in autophagy slows cellular aging and clears away protein aggregates, which decreases the risk of neurodegenerative disease. Disruption of this essential process can cause neurodegenerative disease. Studies on mice have shown that intermittent fasting increases neurogenesis, which is the creation of new brain cells. Another exciting result of intermittent fasting on the brain is that it induces BDNF expression, which increases the resistance of neurons in the brain to dysfunction and degeneration. It has also been shown to protect neurons against the adverse effects of amyloid-beta and tau pathologies and ultimately slow down the aging process in the brain. While there are multiple ways to stimulate autophagy, intermittent fasting is a remarkably effective way and is supported by science. Something worth noting is that despite the endless benefits of autophagy, you don't want too much of it, and you don't want too little of it. Like everything in life, balance is the goal.

OXIDATIVE STRESS

Oxidation is defined as the loss of electrons. The opposite process is called reduction and is defined as the gain of electrons. Our cells are balanced and should be balanced between oxidation and reduction. This process is quite interesting. Too little is bad, and too much is worse. We need this, but, at the same time, it's actually killing us. Like most things, we need a balance. Examples of oxidation that illustrate this process include an apple turning brown when exposed to the air and a nail left outside in the rain that becomes rusty. While this is like what is happening inside of us, we must acknowledge that the process of oxidation can be protective. It can stimulate your cells, kills pathogens, and ensure the proper folding of proteins, which is critical to aging well.

The problems begin when there is an excess of oxidation or oxidative stress. Oxidative stress is essentially an imbalance between prooxidants, or what are known as free radicals and antioxidants. Oxidative stress is the cause of oxidative damage to the cells and tissues which have become overcome by free radicals. This is also called DNA damage which is responsible for accelerated aging.

INTERMITTENT FASTING

While the normal metabolic process produces free radicals, it also produces antioxidants, and optimal health is based on a balance between these two. Most aspects of life contribute to the inevitable imbalance like diet, lifestyle, environmental toxins, emotional stress, circadian rhythm dysregulation, infections, physical inactivity, or excessive physical activity. The next step along this continuum after oxidative damage is chronic disease, such as cardiovascular disease, neurodegeneration, cancer, aging, and an altered immune system. Study after study shows that intermittent fasting reduces oxidative damage, increases cellular stress resistance, and suppresses pro-in-flammatory cytokine expression.[152]

INCREASED LONGEVITY

While more research still needs to be done on the long-term effects of intermittent fasting on longevity, there have thus far been some incredible findings. Most of the studies have been done on rats and mice, but they have shown that caloric restriction has slowed down the rate of aging, increased lifespan, and reduced age-associated diseases. The fasting mice lived longer than the fully fed mice![153] A different study discusses the impact on gene expression and found that fasting can trigger metabolic regulation which expresses the longevity genes, SIRT1 and SIRT3.[154]

It says something about our current health-care system that the first option for most doctors is to recommend a pharmaceutical for just about anything when there is substantial scientific evidence that fasting often results in a greater outcome.

AN EASIER WAY TO APPROACH FASTING

For those of us who find it daunting to go days (or even one day) without food, there is a viable alternative called the fasting-mim-icking diet (FMD). This is a diet formulated by Dr. Valter Longo, a professor of gerontology and biological sciences and director of the

Longevity Institute at USC. He has spent over thirty years studying aging and was instrumental in the discovery of pathways in cells, specifically key genes activated by proteins and sugars which regulate aging. Dr. Longo has found that constant eating prevents our body's innate ability to regenerate our cells and organs. He feels that both the type and the quantity of food are problematic. Dr. Longo confirms what other studies have shown, "that periodic fasting could activate stem cells and promote protection, regeneration, and rejuvenation in multiple organs, significantly reducing risk factors for diabetes, cancer, Alzheimer's and heart disease."

When you buy the FMD, you gain the advantages of a clinically proven diet that mimics a fast without experiencing the hunger of not eating anything at all for five days. In addition to avoiding the hunger accompanying traditional fasts calling for no food at all, the FMD is designed to avoid muscle loss and to optimize hormones, both of which can be adversely impacted during periods of no food. The diet has been carefully designed to contain the necessary ratio of macronutrients, vitamins, and minerals all crafted to make your body believe it is fasting without forgoing all food. It is a five-day, low-calorie, low-protein, low-carbohydrate, high-fat, plant-based meal plan which triggers nutritional ketosis (which is different from a ketogenic diet). Longo's goal is for people to consume low but sufficient protein. I must confess that the data surrounding protein consumption is beyond confusing. Most experts recommend consuming half a gram of protein per pound of body weight. Dr. Longo believes that 0.31 to 0.36 grams of protein per body weight is the appropriate amount. Not only is that a smaller amount but also quite specific! Dr. Longo has found that when you eat more than fifteen grams of protein per day, the process of autophagy is suppressed. The first day is approximately 1100 calories, and days two through five are approximately 700–800 calories. The FMD is available through Dr. Longo's company, L-Nutra, and is referred to as the ProLon diet. He has also developed another fasting diet specifically for cancer patients, but I don't think it is available yet.

The clinical studies are based on doing the diet three times in ninety days to reset your system and then repeating the diet once or twice a year for maintaining your health benefits. It is noteworthy that all of the clinical studies have been done on "healthy" adults, as opposed to those who were already quite sick. "Healthy" is in quotes because while the study participants didn't have severe chronic disease, their biomarkers of health were not optimal. The clinical trials of the FMD showed lowered cholesterol, lowered blood pressure, lowered creatine protein (a marker of inflammation), lowered IGF-1 hormone, which increases the mTOR aging pathway, and reduced visceral fat.

A five-day diet that can reduce inflammation, improve your immune system, and improve your overall health is a worthwhile investment. Dr. Longo explains that these great benefits are due to the restriction of protein and glucose, which allows for cellular repair. When these are both increased, they upregulate pro-aging pathways, such as mTOR and PKA.

Supposedly, people feel energized from fasting because of the use of adrenaline to release stored glycogen and the stimulation of the metabolism. I must confess, I did not experience any burst of energy when I tried the FMD, but I would do it again. There are important considerations involving "refeeding" after the FMD or any fast ends. It is during the refeeding that the cell regeneration occurs, so you want to be careful about what you choose to eat. When you begin eating again, it is imperative to reduce or eliminate processed foods containing flour and sugar. It is recommended to eat only unprocessed whole foods like vegetables, fruits, beans, lentils, sweet potatoes, yams, nuts, and seeds. Ideally, you will introduce one food at a time after the fast ends and make a symptom diary to determine your individual response to different foods. You should not try the FMD, or any type of fast, without the supervision of a registered

dietician, knowledgeable nutritionist, or physician. If you are interested in learning more about the FMD or fasting, there is no shortage of information and testimonials online.

As unpleasant as fasting may sound at first, the reality is that our
bodies have evolved to be able to go without food for many hours,
even days. It is a worthwhile endeavor to approach fasting with the
goal of improving one's physical, emotional, and spiritual health.

MY FASTING STORY

Okay, I thought, why not give this fasting thing a shot? Ordinarily,
I prefer to avoid missing any meals, so the "no food at all" kind of
fasting sounds quite unpleasant. I had attended a conference where I
listened to a presentation about the fasting-mimicking diet and they
were offering a discount, so I ponied up!

On my first day of the FMD, I opened a big box that contained
five smaller boxes, not unlike those popular nesting dolls. Each
box was labeled for each of the five days and contained all of the
food, vitamins, and liquids to be consumed per day. Also included
is a card which lets you know exactly what to eat and when to eat it
each day. Day one has the highest caloric intake, a whopping 1100
calories. While this seemed a bit daunting, I also felt certain that it
was doable. There is a lot of tea to drink each day, which is not too
appealing for me since I find that most tea tastes like dirty dishwater.
I drank it anyway. The day consists of a couple of food-like bars, two
soups, crackers, olives, and a multivitamin. None of the food would
qualify as delicious but neither would it be considered terrible. The
powder-like content of the soups made me feel like an astronaut or,
perhaps, a camper.

Day two of the FMD was like day one but had even fewer calories (750). There were more bars, soup, and olives to eat and more
tea to drink. Day two also had the addition of the "L-drink," which

is a glycerol-based drink intended to halt the breakdown of muscle during caloric restriction. It helped a lot that I was busy and occupied during these five days, so I had less time to focus on my grumbling stomach. So far, so good.

Day three. This day was one of the two most difficult days for me. It consisted of 750 calories, had only one bar instead of two, and no olives. There were two soups, one bar, crackers, a multivitamin, the L-drink, and more tea. I was very hungry today, and I dare say, a tad grumpy.

Day four. This day was better than yesterday. It included not just one but two packets of olives! There was also soup for lunch and dinner, two bars, the L-drink, a multivitamin, and, yes, more tea. I honestly do not know if it was the second packet of olives that I found so helpful, or it was because I was adjusting to the restricted caloric intake. In any event, this day made me less grumpy.

Day five. *No olives today*. I must say that day three and day five were the most difficult for me. Contrary to what I thought on day four, I had not adjusted to the restricted caloric intake. I find it hard to believe, but it must have been the second packet of olives that perked me up on day four. By the way, there are approximately six olives in each packet, so we are not talking about a plethora of food here. Today consisted of one bar, two soups, crackers, a multivitamin, L-drink, and more tea. Had this not been the final day, I am not sure that I could have continued for much longer. Well, I could have continued, but it would have become less pleasant for those around me.

I really don't know if I promoted cellular renewal as the website promises, but I did feel more energetic and clearheaded. In the interest of full disclosure, I did not experience significant weight loss. And when I say significant weight loss, I mean that I didn't experience any weight loss at all.

ACTION STEPS

➤ Consult your health-care practitioner before starting any fast.

➤ Decide which type and length of fast are best for you.

➤ Commit adherence to whichever fast you choose.

➤ If you drink coffee, caffeinated tea, or alcohol, begin tapering the amount down a few days before your fast to minimize withdrawal symptoms.

➤ Drink lots of liquids (mostly water) throughout the fast.

➤ Get moderate exercise during your fast. While excessive exercise is not appropriate during fasting, gentle movements are important for lymph flow.

➤ Be mindful about your first meal after you break your fast. Avoid high-glycemic foods for your first meal.

CHAPTER 15

SUPPLEMENTS:
Micronutrients and Minerals to Optimize Your Cellular Health

MICRONUTRIENT DEFICIENCY

The word *supplement* is defined as something that is added for improvement. It includes vitamins, minerals, herbs, amino acids, and enzymes. They come in different forms including tablets, capsules, liquid, powder, soft gel, and chews.

While the party line among conventional doctors is to obtain your nutrient requirements through food, it is exceedingly difficult to do that today. Dr. Paul Clayton, an expert in pharmacology and nutrition, has stated that "80 percent of us are, in fact, malnourished, due to our still heavily processed diets, which is massively impacting on immunity, chronic inflammation, and more."[155] Many scientists believe

In today's life, we need more nutrients than our food supply can provide. The increase in toxins, both external and internal, the mineral depletion of our soil and chemical-laden food supply, as well as age-related decline in our cell health and our production of digestive enzymes, all combine to leave us unprotected from disease and aging.

that micronutrient deficiency is responsible for nearly every single chronic disease. Micronutrients are defined to include vitamins, minerals, essential fatty acids, and amino acids. They are referred to as "micro" because we only need a small amount. Symptoms of micronutrient deficiency include food cravings, restless sleep, headaches, low energy, unexplained weight loss or gain, memory loss, brain fog, depression, and diagnosis of osteoporosis, heart disease, high blood pressure, diabetes, cancer, or an autoimmune condition. Most doctors and nutrition experts focus primarily on macronutrients and recommend diets based on protein, fat, and carbohydrate ratios. The role of micronutrients is subordinated if considered at all. You can religiously follow a diet with specific ratios of macronutrients and still not achieve optimal health. Even worse, certain diets, while seemingly healthy, can be responsible for your micronutrient deficiency. Examples of these are vegetarian diets, which can be low in vitamin A, and the paleo diet, which can be low in vitamin D. Vitamins are complex, but we do know for certain that each of them is necessary for the functioning of different aspects of our biology. Diseases result from vitamin deficiencies, and while scurvy, beriberi, and pellagra no longer kill people today, other diseases do. Supplements, while controversial, have been shown to improve our response to these stressors and compensate for nutritional deficiencies.

THERE IS A MISCONCEPTION THAT THE SUPPLEMENT INDUSTRY IS COMPLETELY UNREGULATED

The controversies surrounding supplements are many, the first being the misperception that the industry is completely unregulated. In 1994, the Dietary Supplement Health and Education Act (DSHEA) was passed. This act covers both the manufacturing and sale of supplements and specifically requires that no claims may be made about the prevention or treatment of disease by supplements and that they must comply with "good manufacturing practice" regarding product quality. Supplements are not allowed to be marketed for the purpose of treating, diagnosing, preventing, or curing diseases. Additionally, the Federal Trade Commission (FTC) has authority over the advertising of supplements. They require that the ingredients must be listed truthfully, and if any claims are made, they must be evidence-based. More recently, in 2006, the Dietary Supplement and Nonprescription Drug Consumer Protection Act was enacted. This requires that any "adverse event" associated with the use of supplements must be reported by the manufacturer or distributor. This is the same FDA requirement for pharmaceuticals. So, while the industry is not completely without regulation, there is a great deal of room for improvement. The FDA designates supplements as food and not as drugs and is not responsible for regulating either their safety or efficacy. The FDA was designed to look at food additives, chemicals, and pharmaceuticals, and many of the ingredients in supplements are found in nature. The responsibility for the safety and efficacy of a supplement lies with the manufacturer and distributor which is a little bit like the fox guarding the henhouse. If there is a brand-new ingredient used, then the FDA will step in and "review" the ingredient for safety, though not for efficacy. *Dangerous* is the only designation that the FDA uses to ban a supplement. Merely *unsafe* or *ineffective* doesn't rise to the level required for banning.

DETERMINE YOUR NUTRIENT DEFICIENCIES BEFORE SUPPLEMENTING

I hope I haven't scared you away from supplement use yet. The reality is that there are many unscrupulous manufacturers and distributors of supplements that one needs to be wary of, but that is true

Before even taking the first step to purchase supplements, it is best to do some testing of one's levels. There are several tests available to determine your individual level of vitamins, minerals, amino acids, enzymes, and antioxidants.

for every consumer product. The responsibility falls upon each one of us to do careful due diligence when purchasing anything, particularly things we ingest.

I am not a believer in multivitamins despite almost every doctor recommending them. Multivitamins seem like another one-size-fits-all approach. As I have repeated so many times throughout this book, we are all different. It seems most logical to test to find out where and how much you are deficient. That way, you can get as close to personalized treatment as possible. There are companies out there offering "custom" supplements to match your genetic profile, but the science is not quite advanced enough to accurately prescribe in this manner. One day, it will be, but until that day, current vitamin, mineral, and nutrient testing will have to suffice. Keep in mind that blood tests are subject to interpretation and are based on functional and pathological ranges. They are not perfect, but they can reveal information about your metabolic pathways, vitamin levels, fluid and electrolyte balances, mineral levels, and hydration. You should not aspire to the "normal" range but rather what is optimal for you. Learning this information will allow you to supplement for deficiencies and avoid supplementing for nutrients in which you are not deficient.

Nutrients act in a synergistic manner in the body, and one's absorption and ability to utilize a supplement depends upon the availability of other existing nutrients.

SYNTHETIC VS. NATURAL

Ninety percent of supplements are made in laboratories and are processed or synthesized from petroleum, coal, tar, formaldehyde, cyanide, or other chemicals that you don't want to ingest. There are synthetic and there are natural supplements. The body absorbs and reacts differently to different supplements. *Synthetic* means that they are industrialized from isolated nutrients, and they are cheaper to manufacture and more shelf-stable. The word *natural* has lost its intended meaning because it has been manipulated by marketing efforts. While it is supposed to mean that the supplement is not heated during production and contains no added synthetics, the reality is that the law pertaining to a label with the word *natural* only requires 10 percent of the supplement to contain plant-derived ingredients, and the remaining 90 percent can be synthetic. While some people do respond well to synthetic supplements if they are high quality, natural food ingredients tend to have fewer adverse side effects than ingredients that are synthetic and unrecognized by our bodies. While it has yet to be put into practice, there is a new standard for natural supplements called Naturally Occurring Standards (NOS). This certification will indicate that a product is naturally occurring, organic, and free of GMOs (genetically modified organisms) and synthetics. A particularly bad issue with synthetic vitamins is illustrated with folic acid. Those with one or two variants of the MTHFR gene lack the enzyme required to convert synthetic folic acid into a usable form of B9. Without this conversion ability, the folic acid collects in the liver and can become toxic. It is recommended if you test positive for the MTHFR genetic variation, you should supplement with methylated B vitamins to compensate for a compromised ability to methylate.

EXCIPIENTS

Along with harmful chemical ingredients, synthetic supplements also contain excipients and binders. Excipients are supposed to be inert additives that are used to stabilize, bulk up, or enhance another ingredient. The problem is that they are not always inert and can cause adverse reactions. They include artificial coloring, sweeteners, and preservatives. One noteworthy example of an excipient that is widely used and has the potential to cause harm is titanium oxide. It is a whitening agent and is linked to inflammation, oxidative stress, and decreased nutrient absorption. It seems as though a supplement manufacturer would want to avoid a decrease in nutrient absorption but the use of this excipient does exactly that. Titanium oxide is a nanoparticle and is so small that it slips past one's immune system defense mechanisms. It has been associated with allergies, immune disorders, organ toxicity, and has been classified as a carcinogen.

FILLERS

Fillers are used to "fill up" the supplement so they are a reasonable size. They are bulking agents to make the supplement proportional because some ingredients like iodine, selenium, and biotin are so small that on their own, the appropriate dose in a capsule would appear so minuscule that it would hardly be visible. These fillers include artificial colors, hydrogenated oils, starches, and sugars. Two fillers that should be avoided are magnesium stearate and carrageenan. While the science is inconclusive about whether the suppression of immune cells in rats by stearic acid applies also to humans, this substance is made from cottonseed and canola oils, which should be avoided. Carrageenan, which is also found in nut milks and other products along with supplements, is a thickening agent and has been found to trigger inflammation. Another frequently used additive in food and supplements is gelatin. While it is not definitive, it has been suggested that gelatin, which is known to be made from the skin and bone of beef and pork, can also contain diseased organs. Gelatin is frequently used to make the outer layer of a capsule. This form of a capsule, unlike vegetarian capsules made from methylcellulose, can be responsible for side effects because the gelatin used comes from an animal source and can be tainted with pesticides and antibiotics from the animals.

ARTIFICIAL COLORS AND FLAVORS

Artificial colors and flavors have no place in anything that you ingest. If you see FD&C, or Blue No. 2, or Red No. 3 or 40, these are artificial colors added for no health benefit and have the potential to harm. Artificial flavoring is a chemical soup that will not add to your goal of health optimization. If you have any allergies to gluten, dairy, or soy, it will be worthwhile to familiarize yourself with the ingredients which have names associated with these allergens. Two examples are "food glaze" and "hydrolyzed vegetable protein," and both are gluten contaminants. Other ingredients to be mindful of are flow agents, acidulates found in liquid supplements, and disintegrants, which are for rapid breakdown. If you see the words "time release," don't count on it. Ideally, you want the purest supplement possible, unadulterated with other unnecessary or potentially harmful ingredients.

FINANCIAL INVESTMENT

Another consideration is cost. A protocol including supplements can be costly. I heard Ray Kurzweil, the inventor and futurist, speak at a conference about longevity, and he claimed to take 150 supplements a day! He is not alone in his zeal. I have encountered many people—scientists, doctors, and others—who take large daily quantities of supplements.

This is a concept that should persuade insurance companies to incentivize and subsidize taking appropriate supplements along with other preventive measures, but it appears to be a hard sell.

> While it can be expensive to pursue a healthy life, make no mistake, it can be exponentially more expensive to get a chronic disease.

As usually happens when the large corporations take over the smaller companies, the manufacturing process changes. Some of the smaller companies begin with good intentions of avoiding harmful chemicals in their products but once the large conglomerates take over, profit becomes the bottom line. It is best to avoid buying cheap supplements from Costco, GNC, or anywhere. If you decide to invest in supplements, it is recommended to do so with smaller companies that source their ingredients very carefully and have transparency as to what ingredients they use. I am always a little bit wary of the "proprietary ingredient" label. I understand that they have found an effective combination of ingredients that they want to keep secret, but it's hard to trust that their profit motive won't supersede their health-promotion motive.

> There are fourteen giant corporations (including a private equity group) that own nearly all supplement brands. I guess that this is not surprising since the Council for Responsible Nutrition valued the supplement industry at $122 billion in 2016, and other sources have predicted its value to increase to $220 billion by 2022.

FAT-SOLUBLE VS. WATER-SOLUBLE

Some vitamins are fat-soluble, and some are water-soluble. The water-soluble vitamins are absorbed more quickly and are excreted faster. The fat-soluble vitamins should be taken with a small amount of fat (olive oil or avocado, for example) to increase their absorption. One must exercise caution when taking fat-soluble vitamins because they are stored in the body's adipose tissues (fat) and can accumulate. Excessive doses can lead to potential toxicity.

VITAMIN A

And now, onto the specific supplements. Vitamin A is a fat-soluble vitamin that is stored in your adipose tissue and should be taken along with dietary fat. It is known by the familiar names of retinol and beta-carotene. It is an important vitamin that functions as a support for your immune system as well as making antibodies and antiviral proteins. Food sources include sweet potatoes, green leafy vegetables, spinach, broccoli, asparagus, liver, eggs, and carrots. Signs of vitamin A deficiency include dry, scaly skin, poor night vision, dry eyes, infertility, and acne. To illustrate the synergistic effects of micronutrients, one should know that both zinc and vitamin D play a role in vitamin A sufficiency. An appropriate level of zinc will assist in the absorption of vitamin A, and if you are deficient in zinc, you likely are deficient in vitamin A. If you take high doses of vitamin D, you may be contributing to vitamin A deficiency. Excessive alcohol use and protein deficiency impair one's ability to absorb vitamin A. Avoid taking the synthetic form of vitamin A, which can be identified by the names retinyl acetate and palmitate.

VITAMIN B

There are a lot of B vitamins, and each one plays a significant role in our biology. The two main roles that all of the B vitamins play are in energy metabolism and methylation. Additionally, B vitamins maintain the health of your nervous system, turn food into energy, and reduce the risk of cardiovascular and neurodegenerative diseases. They are water-soluble and excreted quickly, so daily use is important. The B vitamins which affect energy metabolism are B1(thiamine), B2 (riboflavin), B3 (niacin), B5 (pantothenic acid), B6 (pyridoxine), and B7 (biotin). These B vitamins are thought of as antioxidants.

B1, or thiamine, improves circulation, digestion, and brain function. Symptoms of B1 deficiency include vision and memory issues as well as shaky hands. Dietary sources of B1 include brown rice, egg yolks, fish, lean pork, milk, whole grains, nuts, and broccoli. As we age, an adequate level of B1 becomes even more important. The synthetic form, which is less absorbable and is made from coal tar, ammonia, acetone, and hydrochloric acid, is called mononitrate and thiamine hydrochloride

B2, or riboflavin, is important for skin, nails, hair, and red blood cells. Symptoms of B2 deficiency include sore and cracked tongue and lips, scaly skin, weakness in hands and feet, and hair loss. Dietary sources of B2 include meats, cheese, egg yolk, milk, poultry, leafy vegetables, and broccoli. There is a connection between the common genetic variant MTHFR and low B2. It is synergistic with vitamin A in that the two together help improve digestive issues, and it also assists in the absorption of B3, B6, and iron. The synthetic form of B2 is called calcium D-pantothenate and is made from acetic acid and nitrogen.

B3, or niacin, regulates blood sugar levels, improves circulation, lowers cholesterol, and positively impacts skin conditions. Signs of deficiency of this B vitamin include tongue soreness, skin issues, diarrhea, and even dementia. Dietary sources of B3 include organ meats, poultry, nuts, whole grains, fish, and milk. This vitamin is critical for both energy metabolism and for your neurotransmitters. It is known to repair damaged DNA and lengthen our telomeres. We need much more of B3 than we do of B2, but this B vitamin can be potentially toxic in excess. The synthetic form of B3 is made from coal tar, ammonia, acids, 3-cyanopyridine, and formaldehyde.

B5, or pantothenic acid, helps stabilize the skin barrier, creates red blood cells, promotes skin elasticity, reduces inflammation, synthesizes cholesterol, and helps to maintain a healthy digestive tract. Deficiencies are unusual because the vitamin is found in so many dietary sources. The synthetic form of B5 is made from isobutyraldehyde and formaldehyde.

B6, or pyridoxine, maintains the health of the immune and nervous system and provides support for nausea during pregnancy. Signs of deficiency include depression, confusion, skin issues, sore tongue, histamine intolerance, and susceptibility to illness. Dietary sources include meat, fish, bananas, beans, and fortified cereal. Dosage is important with this B vitamin because it has the potential for toxicity at high doses. The definition of a "high dose" varies according to the source, but you should avoid a dose above 100 mg per day. Synthetic forms of B6, called pyridoxine hydrochloric acid, are made from petroleum, formaldehyde, and hydrochloric acid. The synthetic form not only is difficult to absorb but also has been shown to reduce the function of B6 naturally occurring in the body.

B7, or biotin, is important for the functioning of fats and amino acids. It also helps with the health of skin, nails, and hair. Signs of deficiency include skin issues, hair loss, depression, and ataxia (loss of control over bodily movements). If you have taken many doses of antibiotics over the years, it is likely that your biotin levels are low. Dietary sources of B7 include cheese, organ meats, eggs, nuts, broccoli, sweet potatoes, and oatmeal. The synthetic form of biotin is called D-biotin. Usually, any vitamin that is preceded with a *D* or *DL* is the synthetic form.

METHYLATION

The next group of B vitamins, B9 (folate) and B12 (cobalamin), along with choline, are involved in the process of methylation. Methylation is a critical biochemical process that adds a methyl group to a molecule. This process regulates the proper functioning of our cardiovascular, neurological, reproductive, and detoxification systems.

B9, or folate, is one of these vitamins involved in methylation. It helps to produce and maintain new cells. Signs of deficiency include gum disease, anemia, fatigue, depression, anxiety, histamine intolerance, and the inability to effectively eliminate toxins. Dietary sources include leafy greens, beans, peas, fortified cereals, and grains. The problem with the fortified foods is that they are fortified with the synthetic form of folate, called folic acid. While most people should avoid processed foods that are fortified with folic acid, people who test positive for the MTHFR variant need to avoid these foods and folic-acid-containing supplements. The reason for this is that if you have one or more copies of the MTHFR gene, your methylation and accompanying detoxification abilities are compromised. The result of this is that the folic acid collects in your liver and can't be adequately excreted, and that gives rise to health issues. It is advised to choose, instead, supplements containing folinic acid or L-methylfolate.

B12 is critical for the normal functioning of the brain, nervous system, and moods, and it helps maintain healthy nerve cells and red blood cells. The symptoms of B12 deficiency include tingling in hands and feet, anemia, fatigue, constipation, migraines, memory loss, and dizziness to name just a few. Dietary sources of B12 are only found in animal products because the vitamin is not necessary for plants. Because of this, vegetarians and vegans are at a higher risk of deficiency and should supplement with B12. Some sources say that it can be found in spirulina, tempeh, and miso, but others say that it is "pseudo B12" and can block the uptake of actual B12. I discovered that symptoms of B12 deficiency are often misdiagnosed as far more serious diseases, and there is a book written about the epidemic of B12 misdiagnosis called *Could It Be B12?* by Sally M. Pacholok, RN, BSN, and Jeffrey J. Stuart, DO. I highly suggest this book as it covers many of the details surrounding B12. The synthetic form of B12 is called cyanocobalamin and is made from cobalt and cyanide. Even though the amount of cyanide is quite small, it seems to me that if there are alternatives devoid of a highly dangerous poison, one should choose them. Methylcobalamin and cobalamin are both the naturally occurring form and are the better choices.

Choline is neither a vitamin nor a mineral and is included in the vitamin B complex family. It affects liver function, brain function, muscles, nervous system, and metabolism. Symptoms of deficiency include impaired lung function. Dietary sources include liver and egg yolks. The synthetic version of choline is called choline chloride or choline bitartrate and is made from ethylene, ammonia, or hydrochloric acid.

VITAMIN C

Vitamin C is the single most studied molecule. Unlike animals, we are unable to produce this vitamin endogenously and we cannot store it either. Vitamin C is known as both an antioxidant as well as a prooxidant. It acts as a prooxidant at certain doses and in the presence of certain other compounds. When it is given intravenously the amount is far higher than can be ingested orally. It acts as a kind of hormesis when given through an IV and has been shown to help with autophagy (the elimination of damaged and dysfunctional cells), apoptosis, and the recycling of damaged mitochondria. Due to its potential for acting as a kind of hormesis, one does not want to take it during the hours before or after exercise as it can block the beneficial effects. This vitamin offers protection from damaging free radicals and cellular oxidation and is vital for a healthy immune system, wound healing and skin issues, cardiovascular protection, and possibly longevity. There have been studies concluding that vitamin C promotes a longer life span and has been associated with far less premature death.[156] It is a cofactor in the formation of collagen and is known for its skin benefits. It is also necessary for thyroid conversion as well as histamine circulation. Symptoms of deficiency include skin or oral bleeding, dry scaly skin, frequent colds and infections, fatigue, sleep dysfunction, and low bone mineral density. Dietary sources include citrus fruits, berries, brussels sprouts, cabbage, red and yellow peppers, broccoli, and avocados. It is synergistic with vitamin E as it recycles E, and it can increase the absorption of iron and aluminum. If you must take aluminum-based antacids, take them a few hours before or after taking vitamin C. The main controversy surrounding vitamin C is the dosage. Some experts are in favor of megadoses and others say too big of a dose can overload the kidneys. To avoid overloading the kidneys, you can divide the doses of vitamin C throughout the day. It is believed that you can only absorb 200 mg of oral vitamin C at a time. In any event, excess vitamin C is excreted through urine, and while diarrhea is a potential side effect of too large of a dose, it is advised to find the appropriate dose by noting bowel tolerance. If you get diarrhea, lower the dose. Dose and absorption vary among individuals and are dependent upon age, stress, lifestyle, and level of disease. While the RDA (Recommended Dietary Allowance) dose is far too low, it is believed that higher doses decrease disease duration as well as viral antibody levels. There are success stories of individuals taking 200,000 mg of IV vitamin C a day to treat particularly serious infections. As mentioned, vitamin C can be administered through an IV, or it can be taken via tablets, capsules, powders, or liquids. Tablets should be a last resort as they have the lowest level of absorbability and are often excreted entirely. I personally prefer liposomal liquid vitamin C because the claim is that its liposomal form allows better cell penetration. The most ubiquitous synthetic form of vitamin C is ascorbic acid. It is made from GMO corn sugar that is hydrogenated and processed with acetone. It lacks the flavonoids and phytonutrients that contribute to the efficacy of the vitamin. The best natural form of vitamin C comes from amla berries and camu camu berries.

VITAMIN D

Vitamin D is technically a hormone. It is a fat-soluble vitamin which is produced by our skin in response to sun exposure. It helps maintain levels of calcium and phosphorus in the blood, promotes bone growth, and affects your immune, digestive, circulatory, and nervous systems. Deficiency in this vitamin is a common problem and has been said to affect 13 percent of the world's population. Every cell in the body has a vitamin D receptor which can influence the expression of many genes. There are three different genes associated with vitamin D. There is one for absorption, one for conversion, and one for transporting the vitamin. If you have variants in any or all of these genes, it can prove to be more difficult to maintain adequate levels. Like so many other aspects of nutrient sufficiency, there is controversy over what "adequate levels" should be. The Vitamin D Council considers anything below 40 ng/mL to be insufficient and connected to disease. Symptoms of deficiency include rickets, bone pain, muscle weakness, cardiovascular disease, asthma, osteoporosis, diabetes, infections, and cancer. There is an emerging belief that vitamin D deficiency may have a connection to hearing loss. Dietary sources of this vitamin include cod liver oil, fatty fish, mushrooms, and egg yolks. This vitamin is not without its detractors and there is no uniform agreement as to what exactly defines vitamin D deficiency or what level is ideal. It is known that an extremely high amount of supplementary vitamin D can be toxic and the ratio of vitamin D to vitamin A is important. Evidently, if your vitamin D is too low, supplementing with vitamin A can be toxic. Vitamin D is also connected to calcium, and for reasons which I'll go into later in this chapter, vitamin D3 should always be taken along with vitamin K2. This is further confirmation of the synergistic relationship among micronutrients and why one should avoid randomly taking supplements. The synthetic version of vitamin D is called calciferol and ergosterol and it is made by irradiating animal fat. D2 is another synthetic form of the vitamin and taking vitamin D3 is preferable. I realize that this may seem confusing, so the best approach is to determine your vitamin and mineral status through testing before taking any supplements.

VITAMIN E

Vitamin E is another fat-soluble vitamin. Its function is as an antioxidant, and it protects cells, other vitamins, and polyunsaturated fats from the damage of oxidation. It also activates certain enzymatic functions and is thought to offer protection from certain cancers and possibly asthma and hay fever. Signs of deficiency include an impaired immune system, anemia, inability to absorb fat, retinopathy, and loss of physical coordination. Dietary sources include vegetable oils (which one should avoid), meat, poultry, fish, eggs, nuts, sunflower seeds, and green leafy vegetables. If one is taking blood thinner drugs, they should be wary of also taking vitamin E supplements. While the toxicity of vitamin E is not clear, it is known that excess vitamin E may cause a vitamin K deficiency and cause blood thinning. Vitamin E is a group of eight separate compounds, four tocopherols and four tocotrienols. The synthetic forms are called dl-alpha-tocopherol, beta-tocopherol, dl-delta-tocopherol, and gamma-tocopherol and are made using refined oils called trimeth-ylhydroquinone and isophytol. These act like toxins in the body and are not easily absorbed.

VITAMIN K

Vitamin K is yet another fat-soluble vitamin. It has long been known for its functions of helping blood clot and maintaining bone density, heart health, and kidney health. It guides calcium safely into bones to strengthen bone mineral density and reduce fractures. It also prevents calcium from accumulating in our vessels and protects our hearts. Recent studies have found that this vitamin is also helpful for glucose metabolism.[157] This vitamin includes K1 and K2.

K1, or phylloquinone, is found in leafy greens, and K2, or menaquinone, is found in eggs, meat, milk, cheese, and fermented soy. The problems with the dietary sources of vitamin K are twofold. One is that the leafy greens have low bioavailability, and it's not feasible to eat the amount of food required to get your appropriate dose of vitamin K. The other problem is that food sources of K2 are quite high in saturated fat, and you do not want to eat the amount associated with the appropriate dose of K2. Signs of deficiency include frequent bruising, excessive bleeding, heavy menstrual periods, osteoporosis, and tooth decay. If you are taking anticoagulant medications (warfarin, Coumadin), consult your doctor before supplementing with vitamin K. You should consult a medical professional before taking any supplements. I have read that if you take statin drugs, the need for vitamin K becomes even more important, but that's one that requires individual due diligence. There is a definite synergistic relationship between vitamins K and D. While one of the functions of vitamin D is to maintain adequate calcium levels in the blood, vitamin K ensures that the calcium circulates properly and does not accumulate in the soft tissues. Vitamin K prevents blood vessel calcification that can result from excessive vitamin D doses. The synthetic form of this vitamin is menadione which is made from coal derivatives and GMO hydrogenated soybean oil and hydrochloric acid. These ingredients are highly toxic and can impair the immune system.

AMINO ACIDS

Amino acids are vital for optimal health. They repair tissues, maintain muscles, increase energy and strength, correct metabolic imbalances, reduce the effects of aging, and are responsible for the synthesis of hormones and neurotransmitters. They are the building blocks that make proteins which, in turn, make white blood cells and antibodies.

The body makes twenty amino acids itself but is unable to make the nine amino acids which are called "essential amino acids." These must be obtained through food or supplements. If only one of the nine essential amino acids is missing, the body's ability to make new proteins and repair itself becomes compromised. The nine which are essential are lysine, methionine, phenylalanine, threonine, tryptophan, leucine, isoleucine, valine, and histidine. As with everything else, amino acids naturally diminish as we age. Dietary sources of amino acids include meat, poultry, fish, eggs, and dairy products. Adequate levels of amino acids will ensure quality sleep, peak exercise performance, the prevention of muscle loss, and the promotion of weight loss. For those people looking to maximize their workouts, branched-chain amino acids play a role. These are three out of the other essential amino acids and are called leucine, isoleucine, and valine. These have the metabolic potential for energy use in the muscles and will prevent muscle loss and increase energy. There are some precautions to be noted when supplementing with amino acids. You should only take them in the short term, no more than six months, and then stop for a period. Too many can be inflammatory, and both methionine and valine have been found to be harmful in excess.

DIGESTIVE ENZYMES

Digestive enzymes are helpful to ameliorate the loss of digestive tract function which occurs with age. If we don't have adequate digestive enzymes, our digestive process is incomplete, we fail to break down our food completely, and we don't absorb all of the nutrients in our food. This can lead to undigested protein, which can trigger inflammation. This is a related cycle in that we need enzymes to get our proteins, we need proteins to get our minerals, and we need minerals to get our vitamins. The three sources of digestive enzymes are our body, the food we eat, and supplements. Most of our endogenous enzymes are made in our pancreas with the balance made in our mouth, stomach, and small intestine. The three types of enzymes that we need are amylase, which breaks down carbohydrates and starches into sugar molecules; lipase, which works with our bile production to break down fats and to absorb the fat-soluble vitamins A, D, E, and K; and protease, which breaks down proteins into amino acids. Some of the foods which are good for enzyme production include papaya, pineapple, mangos, bananas, and avocados. If you are experiencing digestive issues such as constipation, diarrhea, gas, or stomach discomfort, you may want to consider supplementing with digestive enzymes to help predigest carbohydrates, protein, and fats.

MINERALS

Minerals, like vitamins, are cofactors that are necessary for biochemical reactions in our body that keep us alive.

They can also accumulate and must be dosed properly. There are two types of minerals: macro and trace. The five main minerals are also considered to be electrolytes. They are magnesium, calcium, phosphorus, potassium, and sodium. There are sixteen trace minerals, which are also called micro minerals, and they are zinc, iron, copper, iodine, selenium, cobalt, manganese, molybdenum, sulfur, chloride, boron, silica, vanadium, nickel, arsenic, and chromium. Mineral supplements come in two forms, inorganic and chelated. Inorganic minerals must compete with other minerals for absorption, whereas chelated minerals are bound to a protein and do not need to compete for absorption. The words, *glycinate* and *aspartate* are an indication of the chelated form.

MAGNESIUM

Magnesium is the body's master mineral and is involved in over three hundred enzymatic reactions. It is required for fatty acid synthesis, neuromuscular conduction (contracting and relaxing muscles), glycemic control, myocardial contraction, blood pressure, DNA and RNA synthesis, binding serotonin and dopamine to their receptors, activating tyrosine, maintaining ionic gradients, energy production, and bone development to name just a few. Despite the critical importance of this mineral, anywhere from 50–70 percent of the population is magnesium deficient.[158] This is thought to be due to industrialized farming, food processing, the standard American diet, and cellular stress. Magnesium keeps your heart rhythms steady, maintains muscle and nerve function, and keeps bones strong. Signs of deficiency include brittle nails, muscle cramps, PMS, diarrhea, high blood pressure, cardiovascular disease, diabetes, hypertension, osteoporosis, and fibromyalgia. Dietary sources include green vegetables, legumes, whole grains, dark chocolate, nuts, and seeds, but it is no longer possible to get your daily requirement of this mineral from food alone. The synergistic impact of this mineral is illustrated through its relationship to vitamin B6, vitamin D, glutathione, and selenium. One's glutathione absorption is dependent on one's magnesium stores. Magnesium will only be effectively absorbed if there is sufficient B6, D, and selenium. For vitamin D to be functionally effective, there must be sufficient magnesium. Excessive doses of vitamin D can reduce magnesium levels.

There are ten different varieties of magnesium, each known for its own benefits. Magnesium chelate is important for muscle building, recovery, and health. Magnesium citrate is known to be calming, is easily absorbed, and is often used for treating obesity. Magnesium malate is the most bioavailable form and helps

There are many pharmaceuticals which when taken deplete your reserve of magnesium. Some of these include: acid blockers cimetidine (Tagamet), esomeprazole (Nexium), famotidine (Pepcid), nizatidine (Axid), omeprazole (Prilosec OTC), pantoprazole (Protonix), ranitidine (Zantac), and rabeprazole (Aciphex); antacids aluminum and magnesium hydroxide (Maalox, Mylanta), calcium carbonate (Tums, Titralac, Rolaids), magnesium hydroxide (Phillips' Milk of Magnesia), and sodium bicarbonate (Alka-Seltzer, baking soda); antibiotics amoxicillin, azithromycin, cefaclor, cefdinir, cephalexin, ciprofloxacin, clarithromycin, doxycycline, erythromycin, levofloxacin, minocycline, Bactrim, and tetracycline; antiviral agents delavirdine (Rescriptor), foscarnet (Foscavir), lamivudine

(Epivir), nevirapine (Viramune), zidovudine (Retrovir), and zidovudine and lamivudine (Combivir); blood pressure medications hydralazine, ACE inhibitors, angiotensin II receptor blockers, and diuretics; central nervous system stimulants Metadate and Ritalin; cholesterol agents Questran and Colestid; corticosteroids; hormone replacement therapy and oral contraceptives; immunosuppressants; nonsteroidal aromatase inhibitors; osteoporosis drugs; sulfonamides; alcohol; calcium supplements; coffee; and a high sugar diet.

with migraine, chronic pain, depression, sore muscles, and energy. It is found in fruit and wine. Magnesium L-threonate is important for its brain and memory benefits. It improves learning abilities, working memory, and short- and long-term memory and is easily absorbed. Magnesium taurate has heart benefits as well as promoting healthy blood sugar levels and healthy blood pressure. Magnesium orotate is also good for your heart and metabolic improvements. It enhances recovery, energy, and performance. It is easily absorbed and has less of a laxative effect. Magnesium glycinate is good for sleep issues, detoxification, and treating inflammation. Magnesium oxide is the least well absorbed and is beneficial for constipation. Magnesium chloride is better absorbed, but it is made with chlorine. Magnesium sulfate is great for relaxing muscles, alleviating stress, and detoxification. It is the ingredient in Epsom salts.

ZINC

Zinc has received a lot of attention during the pandemic. It is a dietary mineral that is known to improve one's immune system to guard against infectious diseases. There are four different compounds of zinc, and they are zinc acetate, zinc citrate, zinc gluconate, and zinc sulfate. It has also been shown to reduce both the severity and duration of an infectious or viral illness.[159] Other benefits of zinc include improving circulation and boosting energy. It assists in the production of androgens, IGF-1, growth hormone, and dopamine. It is essential to insulin management. It is an antioxidant and anti-inflammatory and is synergistic to the absorption of all nutrients. If you are deficient in zinc, you are probably deficient in many nutrients. It is advised to avoid taking calcium, iron, magnesium, and zinc at the same time in high doses because they will compete for absorption. Zinc has the potential to interfere with the absorption of antibiotics so the two should be taken several hours before or after each other. Zinc and copper have a relationship where the two work together to maintain good vascular and heart function. Too much zinc can decrease copper levels, so they must be in balance. Signs of deficiency include skin issues, poor glucose tolerance, dysregulated hormones, slow wound healing, and hair loss. Dietary sources of zinc include oysters, red meat, cheese, pork, and crab. Sometimes, a diet high in nuts, seeds, legumes, and whole grains can block the absorption of zinc if adequate fermentation or soaking didn't occur with these foods.

COPPER

Copper is a trace mineral, and its role is the formation of red blood cells, energy production, and the functioning of muscles, nerves, bones, joints, and the immune system. It fights off free radicals and inflammation. The appropriate amount of copper is necessary to prevent anemia, histamine intolerance, high cholesterol, and osteoporosis. Too much can be toxic. There are theories that too much copper can cause oxidative stress and contribute to neurodegenerative diseases. Along with zinc, selenium, and iron, copper is thought of as a "heavy metal" and has a higher density than other metallic minerals. Only small amounts of each of these minerals are required by the body to avoid adverse effects. The type of copper that is in cheap multivitamins and in tap water is "inorganic" and is not safe. A copper supplement should have no more than 0.9 mg of copper, and most multivitamins have twice that amount. Zinc and copper have a relationship in that when one is out of balance, the other becomes so as well. There should be an eight-to-one ratio of copper to zinc. Copper exists in places you may not think about like plumbing, cookware, birth control pills, hormone replacement therapy, water, fungicides, food sources, and dental amalgams. These sources contribute to the potential for excessive amounts of copper. Dietary sources of copper include oysters, shellfish, nuts, beans, sesame seeds, lentils, liver, mushrooms, spirulina, and chocolate.

SELENIUM

Selenium is an antioxidant and a mineral known for its connection to immune function, thyroid function, cardiovascular function, and fertility. It is a cofactor in glutathione production, is anti-inflammatory, and is thought to protect cells from free radical damage and lower oxidative stress. Dietary sources include Brazil nuts, walnuts, sunflower seeds, salmon, tuna, chicken, spinach, eggs, and pineapple. Symptoms of deficiency include cancer, digestive issues, and a rise in inflammatory markers. Selenium boosts one's immune response by slowing down the speed at which pathogens replicate and mutate. If you are deficient in selenium, it is believed that you will respond to viral exposure with increased inflammatory stress.[160] Similar to all vitamins and minerals, it is ill advised to look at selenium independently. Each one of these micronutrients impacts the others, and selenium and iodine work collaboratively to improve the thyroid hormone. It is notable that certain digestive issues can prevent the proper absorption of selenium and that too much selenium can cause digestive issues, fatigue, and hair loss.

CALCIUM

Calcium is the most abundant mineral in the body and nearly every cell depends upon it. It is well known for its support of bone and tooth development, and most calcium is stored in the bones and teeth, but it also assists in a variety of metabolic functions. The most important of these are blood clotting, vascular contraction and vasodilation, muscle contraction, and nerve transmission. When your amount of circulating calcium is low, your body draws on the skeleton stores, and the risk of osteoporosis and fractures becomes increased. Calcium has an important connection with vitamin D, phosphorus, vitamin K2, and magnesium. They work very closely together. Vitamin D makes the hormone calcitriol, which improves calcium and phosphorus. If you are deficient in vitamin D, you will not be able to absorb calcium, and you will increase your risk for bone loss as well as lose the functions supported by calcium. It is also important to have optimal levels of these three micronutrients so they don't find their way into tissues where they can increase the risk for kidney stones and cardiovascular disease. Vitamin K2 is responsible for keeping calcium (and vitamin D) out of the tissues and guiding it to where it belongs. Magnesium works with calcium to relax muscles and optimize bone health. Symptoms of deficiency include abnormal heart rhythms, blood clotting issues, muscle cramps, bone loss, high blood pressure, and numbness in extremities. As women age, lower estrogen increases bone resorption and decreases calcium absorption. As men age, lower production of testosterone has a similar effect. A diet low in dairy and green vegetables contributes to calcium deficiency. Dietary sources of calcium include sardines, yogurt, amaranth, blackstrap molasses, sockeye salmon, leafy greens, almonds, figs, tempeh, sesame seeds, broccoli, and beans. Certain medications such as proton pump inhibitors, glucocorticosteroids, and anticonvulsants adversely affect the absorption and metabolization of calcium and can lower bone density.

PHOSPHORUS

Phosphorus is a mineral known to build bones and teeth; filter out waste from kidneys; store and use energy; regulate gene transcription; activate enzymes; assist in carbohydrate and fat metabolism; grow, maintain, and repair cells and tissues; and aid in muscle contractions. Dietary sources include meat, dairy, fish, poultry, nuts, and beans. Deficiencies are rare because this mineral is found in so many foods, even in processed foods. Long-term use of antacids containing aluminum can deplete the body's supply of phosphorus.

POTASSIUM

Potassium is a mineral and an electrolyte that compensates for an excess of sodium. It is involved with blood pressure maintenance, fluid balance, muscle and heart contractions, and digestion. We do not produce potassium endogenously, so we must get it from foods. Dietary sources include fruits, vegetables, lean meats, whole grains, beans, and nuts, with the highest concentration of potassium being in beet greens and beans. The deficiency of this mineral is rare unless one is taking certain pharmaceuticals for kidney or gastrointestinal disorders. There is also the potential for adverse effects from taking potassium supplements if one is taking certain diuretics, certain antibiotics, and ACE inhibitors. You don't want too much or too little of this mineral.

IRON

Iron is an essential mineral whose main function is to transport oxygen from the red blood cells throughout the body to produce energy. It also helps to remove carbon dioxide. There are two types of iron found in foods: heme and non-heme. Meat, seafood, and poultry all provide both heme and non-heme, while non-heme is provided by spinach, beans, enriched grains (rice and bread), and some fortified cereals. The heme found in meat is more readily absorbed but can be hard for the body to regulate. The symptoms of deficiency include fatigue, low body temperature, pale skin, dizziness, headache, and rapid heartbeat. A recent study concluded that both low and high levels of hemoglobin (an indicator of iron levels) are linked to an increase in the risk of dementia and Alzheimer's disease. Specifically, "Anemia relates to a 34% increase in dementia risk and 41% for [Alzheimer's disease]."[161] It appears as though it is the deviations from the mid-range of hemoglobin levels that are associated with the increased risks. While cooking with cast-iron pots and pans can be far more healthy than certain alternatives, if one has an issue with iron overload, they should consider switching to stainless steel, ceramic, or other options.

While most think of iron as a benign micronutrient, Preston Estep, PhD, has researched the downside of iron. He describes the issues associated with excessive consumption of iron-fortified foods and absorption issues that can result in iron overload. Estep points out that when we are young, we need a lot of iron, but as we age, too much iron can lead to an increased risk of neurodegenerative diseases. He concludes that excessive iron can adversely impact one's overall health and longevity by lowering immunity, impairing glucose tolerance and other metabolic dysfunction, and increasing the risk of cancer and cardiovascular disease.

IODINE

Iodine is a mineral and an essential nutrient necessary for the thyroid gland to make hormones. It is not made by the body but is required to control metabolism, nerve and muscle function, and body temperature regulation. Iodine is found in the soils, the ocean, and processed foods. While iodine deficiency is a global problem, the addition of iodine to salt has reduced iodine deficiency in the US and Canada. Other dietary sources include seaweed, tuna, sardines, salmon, lobster, shrimp, dairy, grains, eggs, and vegetables.

Certain foods block the utilization of iodine. They are raw turnips, cabbage, soybeans, and peanuts. Exposure to toxins in our food sources and our environment is believed to also hinder the body's ability to effectively use iodine. Symptoms of deficiency include goiter, other thyroid dysfunction, fibrocystic breast disease, breathing difficulties, fatigue, hair loss, depression, brain fog, weight gain, and cold intolerance. Caution needs to be exercised as prolonged use of high doses of iodine supplements can pose health problems. Excess iodine levels can contribute to autoimmune attacks on one's thyroid gland. Several drug interactions need to be considered before taking iodine supplements.

COLLAGEN

Collagen is the most plentiful protein in the body. We produce collagen endogenously and plentifully until around the age of thirty to thirty-five, at which point our production slows down.

It is made up of twenty amino acids that are known to benefit skin, joint, bone, heart health, and muscle mass. The predominant amino acids are glycine, lysine, and proline. It can be supplemented using tablets, capsules, powder, and liquid forms. Collagen is beneficial to your bones, eyes, gut, heart, nails, brain, joints, ligaments, and skin. In its original state, collagen is a huge molecule and cannot be absorbed or utilized effectively without further revisions. The most effective revision is a technology called hydrolysis which breaks down the big molecule into tiny bioavailable collagen molecules known as hydrolyzed collagen or collagen peptides. These are small enough to be absorbed into the bloodstream and utilized throughout the body. After ingesting hydrolyzed collagen orally, it goes to the small intestine and then is absorbed into the bloodstream where it turns into amino acids and small collagen peptides. Together with vitamin C acting as a cofactor for collagen synthesis, the body produces additional collagen. There are four different sources of collagen supplements. These are bovine-, chicken-, porcine- and marine-derived. Bovine, chicken, and porcine sources are all type II collagen, which is beneficial for your joints and cartilage. Several clinical studies are confirming the efficacy of undenatured type II collagen for relieving joint pain and inflammation and the slowing of cartilage destruction.[162] Marine collagen is a type I collagen that is easier to digest and absorb and is shown to confer many skin benefits. When looking at a label, it's helpful to know that gelatin is collagen in a cooked, more digestible, and absorbable form. There are certain dietary sources that can support the process of collagen synthesis. These include citrus fruits, strawberries, and bell peppers, which provide the cofactor vitamin C; egg whites, tofu, tempeh, cabbage, and mushrooms, which all contain the amino acid proline to help support the growth of connective tissue; beans, kale, pumpkin, and chicken, which are sources of glycine; and oysters, other shellfish, whole grains, beans, nuts, organ meats, dark leafy greens, and cocoa, which are sources of a copper enzyme to help with connective tissue.

MELATONIN

Melatonin was covered in the chapter on sleep, but I will go into more depth about this supplement here. It is a hormone that is regulated by our circadian rhythms and is made in the pineal gland of the brain and cells of the immune system. It has been extensively studied for its many benefits. It is an antioxidant that regulates optimal mitochondrial function. It is well known for its ability to improve immunity, reduce inflammation, and confer both antiaging and anticancer benefits. Additionally, it has neuroprotective, eye health, and mood-balancing benefits. Endogenous production of melatonin decreases with age.

> The amount of melatonin that is secreted is based on light exposure during the day and suppression of light exposure at night.

Melatonin production is heavily diminished from exposure to artificial light at night. The worst hues are blue light and green light. These offending lights are found in LED light bulbs, televisions, smartphones, laptops, computers, and tablets. The best way to circumvent this decline in melatonin production is to avoid or at least decrease nighttime artificial light exposure.

Inadequate levels of melatonin contribute to the weakening of your immune system and make you more susceptible to infectious disease. Supplementing with this hormone will optimize your immune system by stimulating the production and activity of T cells and killer cells to strengthen an immune response. We have learned that too strong of an immune response can result in harm, so what we really want is an optimized, not strengthened, immune system. There has been a recent study suggesting that melatonin can help regulate cytokines and decrease the cytokine storm that is triggered by runaway inflammation.[163] Melatonin is both nonaddictive and nontoxic, and unlike some other supplements, there is no negative feedback loop whereby taking supplements decreases or eliminates one's own endogenous production.

OMEGA FATTY ACIDS

There are several omega-3 fatty acids, but most studies have been on EPA (eicosapentaenoic acid), DHA (docosahexaenoic acid), and ALA (alpha-linolenic acid). The body does not make omega-3s and therefore, it is advised to supplement. The sources of both DHA and EPA are fish, fish oil, and krill oil, but DHA and EPA are synthesized by microalgae, not the fish. The sources of ALA are plant oils, flaxseed, soybean, and canola oils. Most experts advise not using too much of these because unlike DHA and EPA, they lack the benefits of omega-3 fatty acids. The benefits of EPA and DHA include reducing inflammation, cellular oxidation protection, UV damage mitigation, hormone regulation, and cardiovascular and nervous system protection. DHA is known to be brain-protective[164] while EPA is known to reduce depression and cognitive decline[165] and also to lower the production of inflammatory cytokines.[166] Recently, there has been some criticism about omega-3 use. While the sensationalized headlines read that there is no value in these supplements, many articles emerged refuting the findings of the studies and explaining their flaws. The main reason that the studies' conclusions have been rebutted is that insufficient dosing of EPA and DHA was used to conduct the studies. Experts feel that much higher doses are necessary to achieve optimal health. Another important benefit of supplementing with EPA and DHA is the maintenance of the critical fatty acid balance. Due to our poor diet consisting of a lot of processed foods and seed oils, we consume far too many omega-6 fats and not enough omega-3 fats. The current average ratio of omega-6s to omega-3s is often as high as twenty to one.[167] This improper balance is believed to be a contributor to cardiovascular disease, obesity, dementia, and metabolic syndrome. Altering this high ratio is thought to protect against many chronic diseases. Increasing your intake of omega-3 fatty acids and decreasing your intake of omega-6s will both restore the appropriate balance and reduce the risk for chronic disease. Dietary sources of omega-3s include wild-caught fatty fish such as salmon, sardines, mackerel, and herring.

PROBIOTICS, PREBIOTICS, POSTBIOTICS, AND SYNBIOTICS

Probiotics, meaning "pro-biota" or "for life," are quite popular today for their ability to introduce beneficial live bacteria into the intestinal system and to rebalance the gut microbiota. We can consume probiotics through food or supplements. Many digestive conditions are caused by an imbalance of good and bad bacteria in our gut.[168,169] In addition to improving digestion, probiotics have been studied for their ability to reduce inflammation, promote oral health, and decrease allergic reactions. They are live microorganisms that are primarily live bacteria as well as yeasts. They are made up of different species, and different strains are measured in colony-forming units (CFU) which represent the number of viable cells, usually in the range of billions.

Each species and its various strains is unique and confers different health benefits. Once again, one size does not fit all. The probiotic that is making your friend feel great may not be appropriate for you. Taking the incorrect strain can exacerbate your health issues. The health benefits of probiotics are strain specific.

The most common probiotics contain *Lactobacillus*, *Bifidobacterium*, and slightly less so, *Saccharomyces boulardii*. The recommendations are to take probiotics on an empty stomach so that the live bacteria can travel through stomach acid as quickly as possible. The reality is that most probiotics die in the gastric system and don't make it to the intestines. Frequently, only dead bacteria pass through, and while this is certainly not ideal, it is thought that some dead bacteria may be beneficial. Dietary sources of probiotics include yogurt, kimchi, miso, sauerkraut, pickles, and other fermented foods. Another use for probiotics is to protect one's respiratory tract from viral illnesses. Research has shown that probiotics can be protective of the respiratory system and prevent respiratory infections.[170, 171]

There is a distinction between probiotics, prebiotics, postbiotics, and synbiotics. Prebiotics are nondigestible foods or complex carbohydrates like inulin and other fructooligosaccharides which trig-ger the growth of beneficial microorganisms and are used as fuel. They are defined as "a substrate that is selectively utilized by host microorganisms conferring a health benefit."[172] Foods such as onions, garlic, asparagus, green bananas, and chicory root are considered to be "prebiotic" foods. As a result of these fibers not breaking down, they encourage the growth of food bacteria in our gut. While sci-ence is developing on the utility of postbiotics, it's interesting to note that they are the byproducts of the fermentation process from probiotics in the gut. When probiotics feed on prebiotics, postbiot-ics are produced. They are the "waste" of probiotics.[173] Synbiotics are products that combine both probiotics and prebiotics. Recently, a method has been found to increase the efficacy of probiotics. This method combines probiotics with bacteriophages, which are viruses that destroy harmful bacteria while at the same time encouraging beneficial probiotic microorganisms. When the two are combined into one protocol, digestive and overall health improves.[174] There are studies currently to find solutions to antibiotic-resistant bacteria using phage therapy.

GLUTATHIONE

It is a tripeptide, made up of three amino acids linked together. They are glutamate, cysteine, and glycine. Functions of gluta-thione include protecting cells from being damaged from free radicals, apoptosis, and detoxification, improving the immune sys-tem and the transportation of proteins between cells. Symptoms of deficiency include poor immune function, asthma, and other respi-ratory issues. There are several factors that decrease glutathione lev-

> Glutathione is the body's primary antioxidant and is essential for addressing oxidative stress.

els. These include excessive use of acetaminophen (Tylenol), fasting, and low-protein or low-carbohydrate diets. Other causes of decreasing levels of the production and the recycling of glutathione include magnesium deficiency, hypothyroidism, autoimmune disease, poor lifestyle choices, environmental stress, diabetes, insulin resistance, and poor nutrition. There are specific genes involved in the creation and recycling of glutathione, and some people are lacking in these specific genes, GSTM1 and GSTP1. When people lack these genes, they are unable to produce the requisite enzyme that assists in glutathione production. The body does make glutathione endogenously, but certain sulfur-containing foods help increase the production. These foods include cruciferous vegetables, garlic, onions, eggs, nuts, legumes, lean fish, and chicken. Supplementing with exogenous glutathione can be done intravenously, topically, or orally by capsule or liquid. Some believe that oral absorption is not great, but I have read that certain genetic variants put one at risk of using IV glutathione, so please do your due diligence before choosing.

COQ10

Coenzyme Q10 is made by the body and is found in the energy producers of our cells called mitochondria. The main function of this compound is energy production and making ATP, but it also enhances blood flow and protects against oxidative stress. It is also associated with improved cardiovascular, neurological, metabolic, kidney, and bone health.[175,176] There was a study conducted in 2018 showing that CoQ10 supplements were effective in reducing migraine frequency, severity, and duration. The main causes of decreasing CoQ10 levels are aging and statin use. While the use of statins blocks the enzyme which increases cholesterol, they also block the production of CoQ10. People using statins often experience joint and muscle pain because of low CoQ10 levels, and supplementation has been found to alleviate this discomfort. I personally know two people who developed elbow pain while taking statins. I suggested that they both try a course of CoQ10, and, after a short time, both experienced total relief from their elbow pain. There are two forms of CoQ10: ubiquinone and ubiquinol. Most commercial supplements contain the oxidized form, ubiquinone, and it must go through a process of conversion in the body. The other form, ubiquinol, is far more absorbable and has been shown to cross the blood-brain barrier to help the brain.[177] If you decide to supplement with this compound, ubiquinol is more effective. Symptoms of CoQ10 deficiency include low energy, cardiovascular disease, fibromyalgia, multiple sclerosis, and fertility issues. One caveat for people who are serious about exercise is that since CoQ10 is an antioxidant, if you take it right before or after exercise, it is believed to blunt the effects of exercise.

CURCUMIN

Curcumin is the primary bioactive ingredient in turmeric, the spice originating from Southern Asia. This compound is one of the most extensively studied and is an antioxidant and anti-inflammatory. It is thought that its efficacy is due to its ability to suppress pro-inflammatory cytokines and chemokines in several cell types and pathologic conditions.[178] Some of its benefits include its ability to reduce cognitive decline, increase cardiovascular health, lower inflammation, protect existing mitochondria, stimulate mitochondrial biogenesis (the production of new mitochondria), reverse several aging biomarkers, and reduce depression and anxiety. Recent studies have even found that curcumin has anticancer effects because it restricts the ability of cancer cells to extract energy from glucose in the blood.[179] Despite its plentiful health benefits, curcumin is known to have absorbability issues. In its original form, it is not too bioavailable. A great deal of research has been done to discover how to increase the bioavailability of this compound. Two ways to improve absorption that have been found are the addition of piperine, a black pepper extract, and turmeric oil. Some believe that piperine can interfere with necessary enzymes and so you are better off using fermented turmeric for increased bioavailability.

RESVERATROL

Resveratrol is another antioxidant that has been extensively studied. It is a polyphenol found in the skin of grapes, blueberries, raspberries, peanuts, Japanese knotweed, and wine. Many of the studies conducted have researched the benefits of resveratrol on blood sugar control, inflammation reduction, detoxification, neuroprotection, metabolic protection, and cardiovascular protection.[180] Unlike other antioxidants which can blunt the positive effects of exercise, resveratrol has been found to benefit the effects of exercise.[181,182] There are interesting studies on the antiviral potential of this supplement.[183] Several caveats learned from the studies need to be highlighted as this supplement is not without its flaws. Only the active compound in trans-resveratrol has been clinically proven to support one's health. The typical dose recommendation is 100 mg, and it is thought that you need closer to 300–500 mg a day to achieve any benefits. There is some concern that resveratrol binds to iron and may not be safe for those people who have anemia. The studies have not shown that the cardiovascular benefits one gains from drinking wine in moderation are available from these supplements. It is also thought that pterostilbene, which is a metabolite of resveratrol, may be more effective. As with all things you ingest, you should be aware of the potential for adverse interactions with other drugs and supplements.

NAD

NAD stands for nicotinamide adenine dinucleotide and is found in every one of our cells. It is a coenzyme and is critical for converting the nutrients from food into cellular energy. Its main function is to promote and maintain cellular health. Other known functions include improving insulin sensitivity, antiaging, activation of longevity genes, improving circadian rhythms, increasing DNA repair, and the protection of the brain, liver, kidneys, and cardiovascular system. Sirtuin genes are proteins that are critical for maintaining optimal health and longevity and are dependent on sufficient levels of NAD. Our bodies make NAD, but our production declines as we age, and, as we age, we need more NAD than we did when we were younger because of our increased inflammation and increased DNA damage. Each day, our cells experience ten DNA breaks which, when left unrepaired, contribute to aging.[184] NAD has also been shown to protect one from viral infections by preventing viral replication.[185] Low levels of NAD+ are associated with an increased risk of cardiovascular disease, neurodegenerative disease, type 2 diabetes, and accelerated aging. Two forms of vitamin B3, NR (nicotinamide riboside) and NMN (nicotinamide mononucleotide), are both precursors to NAD+. NR is well absorbed in the gut and can boost NAD in cells throughout the body. It also has been shown to slow cellular aging and counteract many of the chronic diseases associated with aging.

NAD stands for nicotinamide adenine dinucleotide and is found in every one of our cells. It is a coenzyme and is critical for converting the nutrients from food into cellular energy. Its main function is to promote and maintain cellular health.

THE CASE FOR SUPPLEMENTATION

The human body can use micronutrients to prevent and reverse disease. While it would be ideal to gain all the polyphenols and other micronutrients that we need from food and beverages, the soil is too depleted of minerals, the food supply is tainted with toxins, we lose the ability to break down nutrients as effectively as we age. Even if none of those were true, we couldn't possibly consume the quantities of food necessary to get all the micronutrients that we need. You still need to focus on a balanced diet, quality sleep, sufficient hydration, and appropriate exercise because these lifestyle choices play an enormous role in the prevention, causation, and reversal of diseases.

THE DARK SIDE OF SUPPLEMENTS

Many companies are entering the lucrative supplement industry today. The barrier for entry is quite low, so we must do our due diligence to avoid the charlatans and the many misleading claims. We cannot be sold simply by the scientific advisory boards on several of these companies. Many of them include Nobel laureates and highly regarded scientists on their scientific advisory boards, but they do not always represent the efficacy of the product. Another note of caution is that many supplement companies "white label" their products. This means that a product is sold under a brand name but is manufactured by a different company. If you see a "proprietary blend" listed in the ingredients of a product, be very wary. This is a way for the company to avoid accountability and transparency. It is not in the consumer's best interest.

It is critical that you choose brands that are free of heavy metals, toxins, and binders. ConsumerLab is a website that provides independent test results and uses evidence to identify the most effective and safe supplements. Certain supplement companies only sell to doctors and tend to be of higher quality. Some of these practitioner companies include Designs for Health, Metagenics, and Ortho Molecular Products. Cold processing is a method that is better at preserving nutrients in supplements. It is also worth noting that your urine color is an indication of your absorption level. If it is bright yellow, you are not absorbing most of your supplements. It is thought that most people only absorb about one-third of the minerals and vitamins ingested. It is best to take minerals at a different time from

In doing your own due diligence, look for third-party certification and CGMP which stands for "Current Good Manufacturing Practice." This will reduce the risk that the supplements have not undergone proper lab testing and medical supervision and will, accordingly, reduce the risk of harm.

when you take your other supplements because they can negate each other. When it comes to the appropriate dose, it is individual, and the goal should always be to take a therapeutic dose to address your deficiency but to avoid taking more than necessary. Paracelsus, born Theophrastus von Hohenheim, a Swiss physician often referred to as the "Father of Toxicology," stated, "Poison is in everything, and nothing is without poison. The dosage makes it either a poison or a remedy."

There are many recommendations of "cycling" or "pulsing" your supplements, and I think it's a good idea to adopt a rotational regime. This can be done in many ways from taking them for two to three months and then stopping them or taking a few one day and then a different combination the next, and so on. Research the potential interactions of any medications you are taking before adding supplements. An example of why this is important is that iron and calcium supplements can affect your body's ability to absorb certain medications. It is rarely mentioned that supplements usually lack the requisite cofactor nutrients necessary to assist in absorption.

Another precaution is that there is a negative feedback loop with some supplements. If you take certain vitamins, supplements, and even hormones exogenously, your body shuts down its own endogenous production. Just because a company has a persuasive marketing campaign or your friends have experienced positive results does not in any way mean that the same supplement will be safe and effective for you. The use and prescribing of supplements are becoming similar to that of pharmaceuticals. They are being prescribed or suggested to address a particular symptom without first investigating the root cause of the symptom. I think this is a misguided approach.

In the future, my hope is that artificial intelligence, other forms of technology, and diagnostics will all collaborate to determine precisely which nutrients we have in our body, which ones we are lacking, and the precise doses to compensate. We will be measuring deficiencies, addressing deficiencies, and measuring again. This will be life-changing as micronutrient sufficiency is essential.

ACTION STEPS

➤ Begin with testing. Have your blood drawn to determine your level of micronutrient deficiency. Do not randomly take supplements because an article or a friend persuaded you it would be helpful.

➤ Choose your brands of supplements carefully with the goal of only ingesting the purest ones.

➤ Look for third-party certification and CGMP on your supplement bottles.

➤ Monitor your symptoms and experiment with the dose.

➤ Adopt a rotational regime, instead of taking all of your chosen supplements seven days a week continuously.

➤ Pay close attention to how you feel when taking your supplements and when you are not taking them.

➤ Only add one new supplement at a time and monitor your reaction, or lack thereof, for a week before adding another one.

CHAPTER 16

GENETICS, EPIGENETICS, and GENOMICS:
The Emerging Field Which Identifies One's Disease Risk

EACH GENE HAS A SPECIFIC job to do. The specific version of every gene that you carry is called your genotype. This is distinguished from your phenotype, which is defined as the observable characteristics of an organism resulting from the interaction of its genotype with the environment and expressed by a specific trait, like eye color. Depending on your individual genotype, you will have a different response to everything. Each gene is composed of smaller molecules that are represented by a combination of letters. These letters are called alleles and are

Genetics is the future of medicine. Genetics refers to the study of genes and their roles in inheritance. We inherit our genes from our mother and our father, unlike our mitochondria, which we inherit in total from our mothers. Genes carry the instructions for carrying proteins which direct the activities of cells and functions in the body.

represented by *A* for adenine, *G* for guanine, *C* for cytosine, and *T* for thymine. *A* binds with *T* and *C* binds with *G*, and they form the rungs on the ladder of our DNA. Each gene consists of two hundred thousand base pairs, and the entire genome is made up of more than three billion DNA base pairs. Each one of us has between twenty thousand to twenty-three thousand genes. DNA stands for deoxyribonucleic acid, and it is a large molecule that stores the genetic code. The difference between two people can be about ten million base pairs. While DNA contains the genetic blueprint and forms a double helix, RNA helps to translate the blueprint into proteins and forms a single helix. This is a fascinating area of science that is still evolving. Currently, only about 1 percent of the genome is understood, but with the use of artificial intelligence, that percentage will continue to grow. As our understanding grows, the price of sequencing will decline. In 1999, it cost $100 million to sequence a genome. Today, the price is around $1,000 depending upon how comprehensive the sequencing is, and this price will continue to decline further to make it accessible to everyone.

Genetic information will be used to personalize medicine, and personalized medicine in the future will result in diseases being diagnosed earlier and more accurately. *Personalized medicine* is defined as "patients' unique environmental influences as well as the totality of their genetic code [...] to tailor personalized risk assessments, diagnoses, prognoses, and treatments."[186] The most accurate way to assess your personal risk profile is to sequence your genome.

Genomics is the study of the entirety of a person's genes, including interactions of those genes with each other and with one's environment.

While the Human Genome Project has been around for over thirty years, genomics remains an emerging area. Science still needs to evolve further. Currently, the main purpose to sequence one's genes is to determine your relative-disease-risk profile so that you can take actionable steps to promote wellness and reduce your risk of chronic disease.

MONOGENIC VS. POLYGENIC DISEASE

I believe that one day in the future, hopefully soon, all babies will be sequenced at birth. In addition to yielding useful information, this will reveal monogenic disorders. A monogenic disorder is a mutation in one gene, such as Huntington's disease for example. While the field studying polygenic diseases is still developing, this is an important area as it pertains to genes that are expressed or suppressed due to lifestyle choices and are responsible for chronic diseases. Most health issues don't have just one gene that dictates your susceptibility. It is the combination of multiple genes and your specific gene variants that determine your overall risk and vulnerabilities.

GENES ARE NOT DETERMINATIVE

Interestingly, our genes account for less than 15 percent of the risk for chronic disease. There is a synergistic relationship between our genome, our environment, and our epigenome. While it must be acknowledged that we cannot change our DNA, it must also be recognized that our DNA is not our destiny.

While we may test positive for certain seemingly scary genes or SNPs, it is not a foregone conclusion that merely having the gene or SNP (unless it's for a single-gene disease, but those are rare), will guarantee contracting the associated disease.

A SNP is a single nucleotide polymorphism or a single base change known as a gene variation. These occur normally in everyone, and, on average, each of us has millions of SNPs in our genome.[87]

THE VALUE OF SEQUENCING

There is an expression which states that the gene loads the gun, but the lifestyle choice pulls the trigger. We have learned that for the most part, genes are not determinative. We can control, to a significant degree, the expression or suppression of our genes by our lifestyle choices.

New genomic tests can quickly identify one's DNA in their blood supply and identify the pathogens which could cause illness. This will greatly advance the field of diagnosis because of the rapid turnaround of these tests. It will be an improvement for the current use of microbiology diagnostics. The cost of the tests and the reluctance of the insurance company to support their use have made them unavailable to most people. While there are still several kinks that need working out, eventually, this form of testing will advance health care and will reduce the incidence of doctors treating patients for what they think they have and instead, treat them for what, in fact, they have.

WHOLE-GENOME SEQUENCING VS. GENOTYPING

These tests have flooded the market in recent years and should at least be credited with raising attention toward the field of genetics and genomic testing. One of the problems associated with these rather gimmicky tests is that they have a high error rate. There have been studies that have revealed that the false-positive rates of disease with these home tests are as high as 40 percent.[188] Not only is there a high percentage of false positives, but in 2019, there was a study that showed that nearly 90 percent of participants of a particular DTC test who carried a BRCA mutation (for breast and ovarian cancer) would have been missed because the company only tests and reports on three of the mutations, while others could be present.

Another problem with these tests is that much of the data you receive is not clinically significant. An example of this is that my niece learned from her test that she has an SNP which predisposes her to a high risk for a unibrow and another for excessive ear wax. While it seems as though both issues are ascertainable without a DNA test, even if they weren't, neither issue requires action.

> There is a substantial difference between having your whole genome sequenced from a university or facility which specializes in this type of testing and the readily available direct-to-consumer testing (DTC) kits. The DTC tests reveal approximately 0.2 percent of your genome and are more appropriately called "genotyping" instead of genome sequencing.

PRIVACY CONCERN

One more problem that I find with these tests is the fact that, in addition to the fee that the consumer pays them for the test and the analysis, the company makes additional money by selling everyone's personal information to drug manufacturers. There is a claim that the data is anonymized, or what is referred to as "de-identified," but it is unclear if that is even possible. This is also an issue with whole-genome sequencing that needs to be improved. The reality is that we don't really own our health data. It exists on servers just waiting to be hacked and misappropriated. Perhaps we should consider owning one's health data as a civil right. In Estonia, people do own their own health data, and if that was true in the US, it might incentivize people to get sequenced. There are methods in place to "de-identify" the patient's data when sequenced, but the laws surrounding health-care data are complex. In 2008, the Genetic Information Nondiscrimination Act (GINA) was passed, and, while it is flawed, it does prevent group health and Medicare plans from using one's genetic data in a discriminatory manner. It also prevents discrimination in employment decisions like hiring, firing, and promoting. Hopefully, in the future, it will be expanded to cover the prevention of data usage for life insurance, disability insurance, and long-term care insurance. There is also the issue of cyber security and the ubiquitous data breach.

BENEFITS OF SHARING DATA

The sharing of health data along with artificial intelligence has the potential to advance science, medicine, and health care. Improved diagnosis, treatments, and prevention of disease will occur sooner when researchers have more diverse data to study. Perhaps we should embrace the idea of sharing our health data to promote the public good. Our understanding of the human genome will advance when more data is available.

An alternative perspective to the legitimate privacy concern is the goal of benefiting society. HIPAA and other protective health-care regulations have made research and data sharing exceedingly difficult.

Technology is by no means a strength of mine, but I imagine that blockchain platforms and quantum computing may help with the protection and the use of giant data sets in the future. In my opinion, the government should subsidize genome sequencing, de-identify the samples, and then turn them over to major universities and research clinics. While there will be costs upfront, the health-care costs saved using the information for diagnosis, treatment, and prevention will more than compensate for any initial costs.

OMNIGENIC MODEL

Yet another issue with the DTC tests is that they simply identify a handful of SNPs, and our biology and genetics are far more complex than that. Looking at genes or SNPs in isolation is a flawed approach. There is an approach called the omnigenic model which views the genome in a way that accepts that nearly every gene impacts every other gene. Our genome is an extraordinarily complex interrelated network and should not be viewed in terms of isolation. Two fascinating examples of the compensatory nature or interrelatedness of genes are the genes increasing one's risk for Alzheimer's disease and the one for sickle cell anemia. The APOE4 gene, conferring a higher risk for Alzheimer's disease, offers protection against parasite infections, and the gene conferring a higher risk for sickle cell anemia offers protection against malaria. I am endlessly amazed and humbled by the complexity of our biology!

OMICS

Related to the field of genetics is the area referred to as "omics." This is defined as the analysis of large biological data sets and covers several specific areas. Some of these areas are metabolomics, dealing with cellular metabolism; proteomics, dealing with proteins; transcriptomics, dealing with mRNA; nutrigenomics, dealing with the interaction of one's genes and food; and pharmacogenomics, the interaction involving medications.

One of the preeminent leaders in the field of genetics and genomics is Dr. Robert Green, MD, MPH. He is a professor of medicine (genetics) at Harvard Medical School and a physician-scientist. Dr. Green is internationally known for his research in the field of preventive genomics and the director of the Preventive Genomics Clinic at Brigham and Women's Hospital in Boston, where one can get their whole genome sequenced. When I first heard Dr. Green speak at a conference, I became instantly convinced that genome sequencing is the future of medicine. I briefly struggled with the privacy concerns associated with this personal data collection endeavor and ultimately decided that it was worth it. The stark reality is that we don't have any privacy left at all, so I felt that the trade-off would be of value. I went to Dr. Green's clinic at Brigham and Women's Hospital and had my genome sequenced, and I now have an enormous file of my sequenced raw data. While it is not exactly useful, I know that as science continues to evolve, we will learn more about our genes and what actions we can take to optimize them. Soon, there will be platforms to run the raw data through to gain further insight. I highly encourage all of you to get sequenced. The resulting data will become more and more valuable as time goes on.

PHARMACOGENOMICS

The field of pharmacogenomics is supported by a great deal of scientific studies and investigates how one metabolizes medications based upon their individual genetics.

As in every area of medicine, one size does not fit all. Most studies on medications exclude children, pregnant women, and some studies have very few female participants at all. The historical reason for this is it is believed that the hormonal fluctuations experienced by women will skew the results. This may or may not be true, but since women metabolize drugs differently than men, they are at a higher risk for adverse effects. The underrepresentation of women in these drugs' clinical studies has resulted in inappropriate dosage recommendations. If you choose to have your genes tested through a company focused on pharmacogenomics, you can learn pertinent information as to accurate doses and specific medication that can be lifesaving. More than 95 percent of Americans have genetic variations that indicate the potential for either an adverse reaction or no benefit whatsoever from common medications. Adverse reactions cause more than a hundred thousand deaths in the US and cost the health-care system $30 billion a year. Approximately one-third of those deaths are caused by gene-drug interactions. The field of pharmacogenomics can inform you of what the wrong medications are for you to take. I suspect that sometime in the future, it will be considered malpractice for a doctor to prescribe medications (with a prescription or without) and to use anesthesia without first knowing the patient's genetic susceptibilities. Aside from the potential of the wrong medications and your genes causing adverse reactions, medications can also cause, among other things, genes to express negatively.

NUTRIGENOMICS

Nutrigenomics is another interesting emerging field. While I don't believe that the science underlying this area has advanced as far as that for pharmacogenomics, hopefully, it will become increasingly more validated. It deals with nutritional factors which influence gene transcription and expression. The goal of this area is to identify the unique dietary factors an individual needs to have the most optimal outcomes.

The diet you choose, or the ratio of macronutrients, should be based on your genes. Certain genetic profiles are better suited for low saturated fat, while others are better for a diet rich in high saturated fat. The same is true for the association between

> Food is information that impacts the expression of your genes. Our genes influence how we absorb nutrients and how we metabolize carbohydrates, proteins, and fats.

genes and high or low protein and high or low carbohydrate diets. For example, those who test positive for the APOE4 gene will have an increased sensitivity to saturated fat and their LDL will probably spike with a high-fat diet. While learning this may be frightening for some people, it does not mean with certainty that having this SNP will guarantee that you will get a neurodegenerative disease. It does, however, give you valuable, actionable information that will inform your lifestyle choices. The knowledge that people carrying this particular SNP have a higher sensitivity to saturated fat allows you to avoid trendy diets like the keto diet. These people will have better health outcomes by eating a Mediterranean diet. Individuals with certain genotypes have a higher risk of diabetes and increased cholesterol when eating an excess of saturated fat, whereas others with different genes may have better fat metabolism.[189] Another example of actionable knowledge resulting from genome sequencing is learning that you carry the MTHFR SNP. It is not uncommon to have this SNP, and it alerts you to your compromised folate metabolism. In response to this awareness, you can choose to supplement with a particular type of B vitamin that is methylated to compensate for this genetic variation. Although, randomly supplementing with methylated B vitamins without a strategic plan illustrates the synergistic nature of our genes. If you have compromised folate metabolism, the result is that you do not methylate sufficiently, which has negative implications. Taking a methylated form of B vitamins will assist in this issue, but you do not want to take too high of a dose because that can cause overmethylation, which has its own set of negative implications, like turning off tumor suppressor genes. This field is particularly exciting because what we eat and how much we eat has one of the most profound influences on our health.

BEWARE OF CHARLATANS SELLING UNVALIDATED PRODUCTS

Unfortunately, there are a lot of charlatans out there attempting to take advantage of hopeful people by promising to tell them exactly what to eat, what supplements to take, and what kind of exercise to do based on their genetic testing. I recently learned of a health coach selling supplements based on her clients' SNPs, and I was stunned. While this sounds like a terrific idea, at this date, no one can create supplements based on your SNPs. I think that one day this will be available, and it will be incredibly valuable for optimal health, but the science is not yet rigorous enough to make validated claims, and there is a great deal of misinformation transmitted today. Knowing your SNPs and genes is critical information because it informs you which lifestyle changes to make to improve your health. Your genetic data will not change, so as science advances, you can apply new discoveries to your data and get one step closer to creating a personalized protocol for your best health outcome.

EPIGENETICS

This term was first used by Conrad Waddington in 1942 to mean "a branch of biology which studies the causal interactions between genes and their products which bring the phenotype into being." This area did not receive a great deal of recognition until years later when the definition was refined to mean "the study of changes in gene func-

It cannot be reiterated enough that knowledge of your genes is not a cause for worry but rather an opportunity for a lifestyle change. The emerging field of epigenetics is the study of how your environment and the choices you make affect the function of your genes.

tion that are mitotically and/or meiotically heritable and that do not entail change in DNA sequence."[190] The Greek definition of the word *epigenetics* breaks it down to define the prefix *epi-* as referring to biological changes that occur that are "on top of" or "in addition to" those directed by our individual genes. Genes can be expressed or silenced based upon our lifestyle choices and our environment. Poor choices can influence genes in a way that results in a diseased state. This is confirmed in the statistic that around 5–10 percent of chronic diseases are due solely to genetics, and the other 90–95 percent are due to environment and lifestyle. Included in these epigenetic influences are toxin exposures, sleep, nutrition (what and when you eat), stress management, emotions, beliefs, spiritual experiences, lack of social connection, and exercise or how you move.

EPIGENETIC TESTING

While epigenetic testing is quite new and the results of these tests should be given only moderate weight, it is an exciting new area. Many companies are selling these tests and the names of these companies can be found in chapter 19; Elysium Health is the company that I chose to try one of these tests. Elysium Health is based in the North East and has a very impressive list of scientific advisors. It is a dietary supplement company focused on age-related issues. Recently, they added to their list of offerings a test called "Index" which measures both your biological age and your cumulative rate of aging. It also gives you lifestyle recommendations based on your results to optimize your aging.

HORVATH DNA AGING CLOCK

Methylation is a biochemical process that, among other things, alters DNA without changing its sequence. As we age, this process of methylation changes and can be a measure of our epigenetic age. Dr. Steve Horvath, a professor of human genetics and biostatistics at UCLA, created an epigenetic clock known as the Horvath DNA aging clock. The clock is based on a biochemical

Epigenetic changes to your DNA are based on your lifestyle choices and your toxin exposure and can influence your disease risk. Epigenetic clocks are predictors of biological age based upon these changes in one's DNA methylation profile.

test using blood or saliva and looking at 353 epigenetic markers to calculate one's epigenetic age. His theory is that DNA methylation regulates genes and genes regulate aging so that this is a better estimation of age. While it is not definitive, the epigenetic clock tends to measure age in a better way than mere chronological age. As we all know, everyone ages at a different rate. One fifty-year-old can be and appear far healthier than another fifty-year-old. You can go online to the DNA Methylation Age Calculator and calculate your epigenetic age. Horvath has stated that "our research reveals valuable clues into what causes human aging, marking a first step toward developing targeted methods to slow the process."[191] Healthy nutrition, physical activity, and higher education have all been associated with slower epigenetic aging while higher body mass index and metabolic syndrome are among the factors associated with accelerated epigenetic aging.

GENOME SEQUENCING VS. GENE EDITING

Genome sequencing needs to be distinguished from gene editing. Recently, gene editing has received a lot of attention in the press. This process uses technology to modify DNA by either adding, removing, or altering genes at specific places in the genome. It is essentially cutting and splicing DNA sequences and has great potential to eliminate or cure disease in the future. It comes at the cost of some profoundly serious ethical implications and the possibility of abuse. Jennifer Doudna, a biochemist and professor at UC Berkeley, is the co-inventor of the technology, CRISPR, used to edit genes. Amidst patent fights and international competition, she wrote a book called *A Crack in Creation* where she describes the paradox by stating, "CRISPR offers both the greatest promise and, arguably, the greatest peril for the future of humanity." One of the many noteworthy aspects of Doudna's invention is that it can alter both somatic and germ cells. Somatic cells are those which are not passed down or inherited by subsequent generations, and germ cells are those which are inherited.

GENE THERAPY

Yet another similar but different gene-related topic is gene therapy. This is not the same as gene editing because it does not correct or remove a defect permanently. Instead, gene therapy involves the use of a viral vector to deliver one or more copies of a working gene to replace a malfunctioning gene that is causing a genetically based disease. If you are interested in learning more about this area, there is a woman named Liz Parrish whom I've heard speak several times about her work in the field of gene therapy. She is the CEO of BioViva Sciences USA, Inc., and is focused on ways to employ gene therapy to treat the diseases of aging. Her story is quite compelling as she has used herself as a guinea pig to test treatments.

While this is a new frontier in medicine, the last twenty years or so have experienced a revolution in genomics which will continue to advance. For the individual, genomic sequencing will identify predispositions to disease, identify susceptibility to toxins, chemicals, and other things we ingest, and it will enable the customization of lifestyle choices. You will be able to take advantage of personalized medicine where the individual patient will be the "n-of-1. " An N of 1 means that you are the only sample and results are specific to you. Diagnosis and treatment will be specific for the individual according to their genome, transcriptome, proteome, and all of the other -*omes*! One day, your sequenced genome will be a part of your electronic health record, and we will evolve from generalized medicine which is based on population averages to a new standard of health care.

PERSONAL STORIES ILLUSTRATING THE BENEFIT OF SEQUENCING

When attending a lecture on genetics and genomics, I heard a very persuasive story about the benefits of genome sequencing of newborn babies. The story was about a newborn baby girl who was failing to thrive. Many doctors became involved with her case and ordered every possible test to determine the cause of her medical issues. Test after test, including some which were unnecessarily invasive, were unsuccessful in determining what was so terribly wrong. Finally, after eighteen months of the baby's steady decline, someone suggested that her genome be sequenced. After doing this, the doctors were able to diagnose her disease effectively and stop any further decline. Had the baby girl been sequenced at birth, much of her suffering could have been avoided. She had a single-gene disease, which is rare but if diagnosed early can be treated more effectively and avoid the need for useless tests.

While the story of the baby is about a single-gene disease, the next story has more application to the general population because it deals not with a monogenic disease, but rather with a particular SNP or gene variant that can predispose someone to a higher risk of disease. This story is about a man who learned that his sister nearly died of a pulmonary embolism. His sister's job required her to fly a great deal, and she always remained in her seat and worked on her laptop during the entire flight. At the end of one of these flights, she experienced a severe health crisis that could have been the end of her life. Her brother, who told me this story, was so disturbed by the near loss of his sister that he was inspired to investigate his own health. One of these methods of investigation was getting his genome sequenced. Among other things, he learned that he had a particular gene variant that predisposed him to a higher risk of getting blood clots. After learning this, both he and his sister made certain that they always wore compression garments while flying. They were able to take action to reduce their risk based on their individual genetic information. I think that both stories illustrate how powerful information is and the ways to make use of it. Having your genome sequenced is like learning about your personal operating system, and that will be enormously beneficial.

LAURIE'S STORY

Laurie's story of survival is truly remarkable. Fifteen years ago, she learned that she had pancreatic cancer. After living for fifty-five years in excellent health, she was faced with a diagnosis of a cancer that had a particularly grim prognosis. Statistically, 94 percent of all patients with pancreatic cancer die within twelve months of diagnosis. Pancreatic cancer is the third deadliest cancer, with no early detection markers.

Throughout her grueling experience, no one ever suggested genetic testing to Laurie. Currently, treatment guidelines for pancreatic cancer state that all patients should undergo germline and somatic genetic testing. Robert Nussbaum, MD, the chief medical officer of Invitae, a medical genetics company, states that "complete genetic information impacts prognosis, precision therapy selection, clinical trial qualification and surgical decisions." Germline testing reveals genetic changes in the cells and includes any changes one has from conception. Somatic sequencing looks at alterations in DNA within a tumor. Germline mutations occur before conception and are usually, but not always, passed down from a parent at birth while somatic mutations occur after conception and are not passed down from a parent. Despite these guidelines, less than 20 percent of patients get genetic testing. This kind of testing can inform as to the cause of the cancer, whether any hereditary risks exist, and also which treatment options will result in the most positive outcome.

Today, Laurie is not only a fifteen-year survivor, but she is thriving. Despite her wonderful outcome, she feels that knowledge is power, and she would have liked to have been offered the opportunity for genetic testing. She has embarked on a career of motivational speaking and cancer coaching. She encourages others with a cancer diagnosis to get genetic testing to help them make more informed decisions about their individual treatment strategies.

Genomics must be available to everyone, not just those who can afford it. Insurers and policymakers must collaborate to make this widespread. A global genomics initiative should emerge because the larger and more complete the genetic data sets, the more effective the outcome. The power and success will be a result of the combined total of sequenced genomes.

GLOBAL GENOMICS INITIATIVE

Genomics must be available to everyone, not just those who can afford it. Insurers and policymakers must collaborate to make this widespread. A global genomics initiative should emerge because the larger and more complete the genetic data sets, the more effective the outcome. The power and success will be a result of the combined total of sequenced genomes. To achieve maximum potential, there will need to be a convergence among science, business, and law. Unfortunately, the current state of the US is sorely lacking in science and technology. It appears that China will prevail in genomics.

ACTION STEPS

- ➢ Consider getting your genome sequenced.
- ➢ Try an epigenetic test.
- ➢ Learn about your personal genetic variants.
- ➢ Consider doing a test for pharmacogenomics to avoid taking medications that can adversely affect you.
- ➢ After gathering this useful information, make lifestyle adjustments to optimize your individual genetic profile.

CHAPTER 17

TESTING and TRACKING: You Can't Fix What You Don't Measure

ABOUT TWELVE YEARS AGO, I found myself in a constant state of exhaustion. I could log a solid nine hours of sleep every night, wake up tired, and need to take an hour's nap every afternoon. When I say "nap," I don't mean a little catnap, but rather, full-out sound asleep. I thought my persistent fatigue was due to driving my two sons to hockey practice and games all over Southern California. I was driving hundreds of miles a week in soul-crushing traffic. Eventually, both of my sons aged out of youth travel hockey, and I was dismayed to find myself still tired! No longer able to blame my exhaustion on driving, I began to look further for an explanation. Thus began my obsession with testing and tracking.

As I have mentioned previously, there is a great expression that says, "you can't manage what you can't measure." When you are pursuing optimal health, your symptoms speak volumes and help identify what you want to treat. Unless you determine the source of your symptoms, you will merely be masking the symptoms and not eliminating the problem. There are two ways of identifying the root cause of ailments in medicine: one is a visual physical exam; the second is by using more advanced or molecular diagnostic assessments. Roughly 70 percent of all medical treatments are driven by one of these diagnostic assessments. The challenge is that symptom-based diagnostics have an extremely low accuracy rate and can delay effective treatment.

Allopathic medicine focuses primarily, if not exclusively, on symptom management.

> Functional or holistic medicine focuses on the root cause, and the determination of the root cause and an in-depth investigation is necessary. The best means of investigating is testing.

There are many different types of tests depending upon how in depth you wish to go. I love quantitative data and am delighted with the ability to collect this data with testing and tracking. There are more ways to obtain actionable information about your biology in today's world than ever before. I have learned both amazing and startling things about my health that I would never have known had I not done extensive testing. I realize that you may not want to incur the costs involved with testing because insurance policies do not always cover the associated costs. This is because insurance companies do not acknowledge the benefit of this valuable information. If your budget does not allow extensive testing, then at least do blood work which is covered by most insurance policies. If your budget does allow, I encourage you to try at least some of the available tests because there is no greater investment than your health. You want to consider your health an investment instead of an expense.

There are two types of testing: laboratory testing and do-it-yourself-at-home testing. Some of the at-home tests gather data by testing breath, saliva, stool, or urine. Other modes of testing obtain data using technological devices.

CURRENT BIOMARKERS CAN PREDICT AND PREVENT FUTURE DISEASE

Most people have at least some familiarity with blood tests. These are critical in monitoring your health status because you can lead a healthy life involving exercise, good sleep hygiene, stress reduction, and good nutrition and be unaware of underlying issues like vitamin deficiencies, inflammation, and hormonal imbalance. While blood tests are not without error, they can give you a snapshot of both your current health status and a forecast of your future health if specific patterns appear. That's helpful because it provides us with the opportunity to turn the ship around before it is too late. An example of this is testing markers (HbA1c and blood glucose) relating to blood sugar regulation. These tests will alert someone in the prediabetes category and give them critical information to alter their lifestyle to prevent prediabetes from evolving into diabetes.

THE PROMISE AND FAILURE OF BLOOD WORK

If I could, I would have my blood drawn every month. I was disappointed with the collapse of Theranos. While the story of the failure of that company is filled with intrigue, greed, and hubris, it highlighted the need for inexpensive and fast-turnaround blood work. I hope that some other brilliant science innovator will continue the mission of this company. The preventive nature of blood work is of great value. But it must be pointed out that there is limited utility in this testing. Most conventional doctors rely on blood work in isolation for diagnosis, and I believe this is misguided. Often, disease or dysfunction is due to many factors. An annual blood test administered by your primary care provider, whether it is a complete blood count (CBC) or one isolated biomarker, is merely a snapshot of the exact moment the blood is drawn and can vary according to many factors. What, when, and how much you ate, what you drank (alcohol or caffeine), how well or poorly you slept, whether you exercised, your level of stress, time of day, and certain medications (prescription and over the counter) that you took before the blood draw can influence the results. All of these actions can cause false positives and false negatives. Fasting for eight to ten hours before the blood work and avoiding all but necessary medications can reduce skewed results.

In addition to the fact that your blood data is constantly changing according to your nutrition, stress, sleep, and other factors, another big problem with relying too heavily on blood work is the issue of laboratory reference ranges and "standard lab values." These ranges are not especially useful because they fail to consider the many variables of everyone and because different laboratories use different equipment and testing methods. First, the range is an average value of the population tested or a "healthy population." The reality is that it is not clear how the "health" of this population is defined and if they are devoid of any disease. Second, the range is the same for everyone without regard to gender, age, ethnicity, or genetic individuality.

This is a one-size-fits-all metric, and one size fits all, while typical of our current health-care system approach, is just not that useful. That is like a one-size-fits-all sweater. Often, the one-size-fits-all sweater fits no one! These blood values vary and are continuously changing, so one must view them as merely a point of reference and not definitive. The term "reference limit" indicates the upper and lower extreme of the reference interval. The term "reference range" is the difference between the two values.

While this metric has some utility, it cannot be relied on exclusively because a result within the "normal" range does not necessarily mean a lack of disease. A consequence outside of the "normal" range does not necessarily mean there is the presence of disease.

No two people are the same, and what is right for one person may not be suitable for you. I don't know what "normal" is, and I certainly do not want to be normal. I strive for "optimal," and I think you should too.

It turns out that even the term "health" is a relative term and can't be considered an absolute state. Health may be defined differently in different countries, the same country, or the same individual at other times.[192] The best way to circumvent these issues is to avoid looking at one blood test in isolation. Instead, add it to various metrics, including other lab results, other testing, and how you feel. You can also repeat blood tests a few times and interpret your results relative to other tests, use an average of all tests, or watch the trends. Despite these drawbacks, I still believe that blood tests should be a component of one's preventive care plan. They are a helpful tool revealing data and metrics that indicate present and future risk factors and the beginning of disease and inform necessary lifestyle adjustments.

"Normal" is relative and situational. Reference ranges differ among populations. My view is that blood lab results "within range" are relatively meaningless because you do not want to be aligned with a mysterious average population. But, instead, you want what is optimum for you as an individual.

The basic blood work ordered by a conventional doctor includes:

- CBC—Complete Blood Count. This is the test that you always hear a doctor on a medical TV drama request! It usually is part of a routine physical examination and reveals the different types of blood cells: red blood cells (RBCs), platelets, and white blood cells (WBCs). It also covers hemoglobin, hematocrit, mean corpuscular volume (MCV), mean corpuscular hemoglobin (MCH), and immune cell differential count. This test can indicate the presence of infection, anemia, and other blood and bone marrow conditions.

- Lipoprotein Panel. This test evaluates your total cholesterol, triglycerides, HDL cholesterol, LDL cholesterol, total cholesterol/HDL ratio, and LDL particle size. This panel measures the healthy and unhealthy fats in the body. It will give you insight into your cardiovascular, stroke, and metabolic syndrome risk factors.

- BMP—Basic Metabolic Panel. This test is used to identify diabetes and kidney disease. It looks at glucose levels, electrolyte and fluid balance, and kidney function. This test measures calcium, carbon dioxide, chloride, creatinine, glucose, potassium, sodium, and blood urea nitrogen, or BUN.

- Hepatic Function Panel. This test measures liver function and looks at blood levels of total protein, albumin, bilirubin (total and direct), and liver enzymes: ALT (alanine aminotransferase), ALP (alkaline phosphatase), and AST (aspartate aminotransferase).

- Comprehensive Hormone Panel. This test measures sex hormones including DHEA-S, estradiol (E2), estrogen, progesterone, testosterone (free and total), pregnenolone, FSH, LH, and sex hormone binding globulin (SHBG); stress hormone, cortisol, and thyroid hormones including TSH, T3, free T3, T4, free T4, and thyroid peroxidase.

ADDITIONAL BLOOD TESTS

While the following tests are not part of a standard protocol, I believe they are of great value, and you should include them in pursuit of optimal health. They include fasting insulin, which will alert you as to your level of insulin sensitivity or insulin resistance. Other tests are hemoglobin A1c, prostate-specific antigen (PSA) for men, IGF-1, C-reactive protein, homocysteine, vitamin D, all of the B vitamins, folate, iodine, copper, zinc, magnesium, iron, ferritin, CoQ-10, and fatty acids (omega-3 and omega-6).

LABORATORIES FOR BLOOD WORK

There are fifteen thousand clinical labs in the US. The website www.meenta.io is an online platform that aggregates the widest array of testing products and laboratory services combined with scientific expertise and clinical oversight. I suggest that you use this as a resource.

It's best to check with your health-care provider for the lab they work with most often. Insurance providers partner with various laboratories; check with your insurer.

Please see chapter 19 for a list of labs.

DIRECT-TO-CONSUMER TESTS

A recent phenomenon allows for the consumer to order blood work directly online without the added step and expense of a doctor's referral. Most of these allow you to go to a lab, have a phlebotomist come to your house to draw your blood, or some even require only a finger prick which you can do yourself.

A list of some of these can be found in chapter 19.

OTHER KINDS OF TESTING

There is no end to the things you can test! While I may not have tried everything, I have tested many, many aspects of my biology. Some of these seemingly obscure tests include:

Food intolerances and sensitivities.

Allergies.

Heavy metal toxicity.

Nutrient deficiencies.

Mineral deficiencies.

Visual contrast sensitivity test (tests for biotoxin exposure).

BMI (body mass index).

Total body water composition.

Comprehensive stool analysis (gastrointestinal health).

GI screen antigen (parasites, yeast).

SIBO (small intestinal bacterial overgrowth).

Gluten sensitivity, reactivity, and celiac disease.

Organic acids test.

MTHFR and other gene variations.

CIRS (chronic inflammatory response syndrome).

MELISA (dental materials reactivity test).

Oral DNA (measures eleven types of bacteria known to cause gum disease and increase disease risk).

Sleep apnea test (tests pathological breathing disorders).

DUTCH test (a favorite of mine): This test is a urine test which is an excellent complement to a blood serum hormone test. It measures one's hormonal metabolites. I highly recommend this test for a complete picture of your hormones.

NEUROTRANSMITTER TESTING

Neurotransmitters are chemical messengers that carry messages from one nerve cell to another. Neurotransmitters regulate the function of heart rate, breathing, sleep cycles, digestion, mood, concentration, appetite, and muscle movement. The different types of these chemical messengers include "excitatory," "inhibitory," and "modulatory." Some of the causes of neurotransmitter imbalance include chronic stress, poor nutrition, and lack of exercise. You want your neurotransmitters to be balanced to avoid diseases like Alzheimer's disease, Parkinson's disease, depression, and anxiety. A list of relevant neurotransmitters includes GABA, serotonin, glycine, glutamate, histamine, PEA, epinephrine and norepinephrine, dopamine, and acetylcholine.

GUT AND MICROBIOME TESTING

Gut and microbiome testing is a relatively new phenomenon and can yield interesting and useful data, while not foolproof. These tests gather data through the collection of stool, urine, and breath. Genova Diagnostics has a test called GI Effects. This test gives you insight into your infection status, inflammation status, and gut imbalances. It shows you your microbial diversity and reveals the metabolic aspects of your gastrointestinal microbiome. This fascinating new area of science merits caution when choosing a testing company. You should be cautious about some of the companies entering this marketplace. The barrier for entry appears to be low, and therefore, some of them are promising things that are not validated by science. Genova Diagnostics and Doctor's Data are two highly regarded companies that, so far, have not committed any malfeasance.

HORMONE AND GENETIC TESTING

I have discussed the different methods of hormone testing in detail in chapter 10. I want to reiterate how useful I find this type of testing. Hormones are critical to every biological function. They affect blood sugar regulation, immune system function, and energy production, not to mention general well-being. I discussed genetic testing in detail in chapter 16. I know that genome sequencing will have the single most significant impact on our health care in the future. I can only hope that the future arrives soon!

BLOOD PRESSURE TESTING

Doctors measure your blood pressure on every visit; this is part of federal law designed to emphasize disease prevention. This law needs to be expanded dramatically. Hypertension or high blood pressure can lead to other severe health conditions like cardiovascular disease and stroke. When measuring, the first reading indicates the amount of pressure put on the walls of your blood vessels. These vessels carry blood and oxygen to your organs with each heartbeat called systolic pressure and it is the top number on the reading. The second reading is the force created when your heart rests in between beats. This is called the diastolic pressure and it is the bottom number. There is a gradual progression from healthy blood pressure to high blood pressure, hence the name "silent killer." For those of you who don't visit your doctor often, it would be beneficial to invest in an at-home blood pressure monitor and monitor this marker at home. Low blood pressure or hypotension is usually not a sign of a problem unless it is abnormally low, and then it needs to be monitored.

RESTING HEART RATE

Science correlates an increased heart rate with an increased rate of mortality. Your heart rate, also known as your pulse, is the number of times your heart beats per minute, and it changes throughout the day. You can measure it at any time. Measure your resting heart rate when you are sitting down, lying down, or relaxing. It measures your heart, blood, and tissues' integrity and health as well as your nervous and hormonal system. It can easily be done at home or anywhere by placing two fingertips on your wrist or carotid artery in your neck and counting the number of beats for thirty seconds and multiplying by two. A heart rate between eighty and one hundred is acceptable for adults, but you want to be at the lower end of the range.

PEAR VS. APPLE SHAPE: WHICH ARE YOU?

Measuring body mass index, BMI, was once considered by the medical establishment to be the standard for testing health metrics. In recent years, research has shifted to conclude that BMI is both an inaccurate and incomplete measure of your health.

A pear-shaped body is one where the fat is located on the hips and thighs and is considered to be healthier. The amount of extra fat you are carrying, and where that extra fat is located, are both critically associated with health risks. A large waist circumference is associated with an elevated risk of cardiovascular disease and death. Ideally, your waist should measure less than half your height. You can easily measure your waist size at your belly button with a cloth measuring tape and compare it to your hip size to obtain the waist-to-hip ratio.

A post from the Harvard Health Blog concludes that while it may be somewhat useful to know your BMI, you must recognize that this number fails to identify any illness. The author of the post, Robert H. Shmerling, MD, states that "plenty of people have a high or low BMI and are healthy and, conversely, plenty of folks with a normal BMI are unhealthy."

HEALTH-CARE TECHNOLOGY

This exciting time of innovation is responsible for the availability of many technological devices which can both promote and track health. The term "biometrics" describes the merger of science and technology to analyze biological data. The outcome of this merger is an attempt to simplify the complexity of our biology.

What was once the realm of science fiction is now becoming mainstream in wearables and tracking devices. Ideally, these devices will be tested in clinical trials and regulated with careful consideration to increase wide-scale acceptance. While they have enormous potential for beneficial contributions to health, there are nefarious actors and companies in the world of commerce, so you must always do your due diligence before buying or relying on these devices. The combined use of machine learning, artificial intelligence, and engineering will continue to give us the ability to track and collect data that will teach us about our biology. When these are in use, we will be able to make observations and learn things that conventional doctors cannot make. The design, functionality, and ability to collect and analyze the new devices have all improved significantly over the last five years and presumably will continue to do so. These devices include heart rate monitors, fitness trackers, sleep trackers, smartwatches, stress level monitors, and other wearable sensors to name just a few. They allow you to see the impact of which foods you eat. They monitor diabetes, chronic obstructive pulmonary disease, and hypertension; measure oxygen saturation and blood glucose; analyze your body composition; detect atrial fibrillation; measure heart rate and respiratory rate; and gather a great deal of other valuable health data. The exciting and positive contribution of these devices will help advance health care in gathering precise, personalized results that will aid in prevention. My hope is that insurance companies will realize and accept these devices' implications and make them accessible to everyone.

These sensors, wearables, and data collection devices are consumer-focused. They will allow the consumer to monitor his health and keep track of this critical data. Many of these devices pair with a smartphone app and transmit the data to one's physician, if desired. I believe this growing area of health technology will incentivize good habits and behavior, but there remain issues of quality and security/privacy. Recently, the SMARTWATCH Data Act was introduced.

This legislation aims to improve privacy protection for consumer health data and prevent the sharing and sale of health data collected through devices and apps without consumer consent. The acronym SMARTWATCH stands for Stop Marketing And Revealing The Wearables And Trackers Consumer Health. I came across a letter sent to Alex Azar by US Senator Amy Klobuchar when Azar was the Health and Human Services secretary. The letter illustrated the concern about Halo, a fitness tracker which sent body photos and voice recordings to Amazon's servers. Halo has been collecting a great deal of sensitive health and personal information and neglecting to protect the privacy and security of this information. There is still a lot to be done in this emerging area.

MY FAVORITE DEVICES

My two favorites of these devices are the continuous glucose monitor and the Ōura Ring. The continuous glucose monitor (CGM) is something that I believe will become a standard of care for everyone in the future, not just for diabetics. While this device is currently part of diabetes care, it is extraordinarily useful for those who don't have diabetes. A CGM is an FDA-approved wearable device that uses a sensor placed under your skin (belly or upper arm) and measures and records your blood sugar levels throughout the day and night, hence the name "continuous." These devices deliver real-time data and do not require finger-stick calibration. They last for about ten to fourteen days and are excellent tools for managing your blood sugar and motivating the reduction of your A1c marker. I was inquisitive about my response to different foods, so I asked a physician for a CGM prescription. I found a tutorial online to self-administer the device onto my upper arm and I wore it for the requisite two weeks. I downloaded an app on my phone to see the collected data, and I learned useful information. Seemingly benign foods like carrots or bananas can trigger dramatically different responses in different people. When some people eat either a carrot or a banana, they may spike glucose depending on their individual physiology. This is critical information to have as it indicates that certain foods are incompatible with your biology. I talked to a fellow biohacker who learned from his CGM that eating popcorn triggered a spike in his glucose. He had no idea that this food affected him in this way, and he adjusted his nutritional habits and stopped eating popcorn. Other people can eat the same food and have no response at all. This is especially useful data, and I think everyone should try out a CGM for at least one fourteen-day period to learn about their response to food. I believe so strongly in the value of this device that I think that everyone will have one of these devices implanted into them one day in the future. Different versions of CGMs are listed in chapter 19. I have read about new startups entering this market, but it may be best to begin with the tried-but-true manufacturers.

My second favorite device is the Ōura Ring. I mentioned it briefly in the chapter on sleep because its primary function is to track one's sleep metrics. This health and fitness wearable and smart ring is made by a company based in Finland. It is not inexpensive at $299, but you can usually find a $50 discount code. Upon purchase, the company sends you a sizing kit to ensure proper fit. This is a smart ring with internal sensors that provides personal insight into sleep and overall health. It tracks sleep states, heart rate, respiratory rate, heart rate variability (HRV), and body temperature while sleeping. It also tracks your activity level in total caloric burn, steps taken, training frequency, training volume, and recovery time. Like so many other things today, you download an app so you can view the collected data. One of the aspects I love most about this device is that it establishes your baseline metrics. This is something that all devices (and even doctors) should do. Unlike conventional blood work and a great deal of medicine today, the data is not based on a "reference range" from "average" people. Instead, the data reported is based on variations from your individual baseline. The ring adjusts to your habits and patterns as you wear it consistently. At the end of each week, I get a notification of my "weekly report." I find this quite useful as it reveals key insights about my past week's readiness, sleep, and activity level.

As of July 2020, Ōura Ring announced a partnership with WNBA (the Women's National Basketball Association).[193] The press release stated, "The Ōura Ring is one of the only mainstream consumer health wearables that measures body temperature directly from your skin rather than estimating it from your external environment. Temperature is a vital component of accurate sleep analysis, athletic performance, and the ability to uncover potential signs of illness."

That last-mentioned feature alone is compelling enough to convince most people of the inherent value of this device. When pursuing optimal health, one should know their potential signs of illness. While I don't believe that the Ōura Ring has been the subject of any clinical studies and, therefore, should be relied on accordingly, at the very least, this device is a great method of evaluating different key metrics. The adopters of this device are a broad group, including NASCAR drivers and Prince Harry!

METABOLIC TRACKING DEVICE

Merav and Michal Mor, twin sisters, both with PhDs in physiology, have developed a small portable device that pairs with a smartphone to measure your metabolism accurately. This device, called Lumen, has been scientifically validated to meet the gold standard for metabolic measurements. It works by breathing into the device and then measuring the ketone levels in your breath, determining whether you are burning carbohydrates or fat for energy. This device aims to give you data about your metabolism so you can take action to become metabolically flexible. Metabolic flexibility is critical to achieving steady glucose levels, a stronger immune system, improved sleep, optimized energy, and an overall lower risk of developing chronic disease. You could probably gather similar data far less expensively by using ketone test strips, ketone blood tests, or keto breath tests. The accompanying app that comes with the $299 purchase of this device will customize nutritional and fitness goals and provide an excellent resource for health-related information.

SMART SCALES

As though it wasn't daunting enough to stand on a scale and see the measure of pounds staring back at you, an entirely new type of scale has been developed to give you more data than you ever thought you needed to know! These smart scales measure your body weight, your body fat percentage (BFP), your body mass index (BMI), muscle mass percentage, body water percentage, bone mass, basal metabolic rate (BMR), protein rate, metabolic age, visceral fat index, subcutaneous fat, fat mass, muscle mass, and protein mass. These scales sync with apps and record and track your data and progress (or lack thereof!). A list of companies making these smart scales can be found in chapter 19.

ADDITIONAL DEVICES AND TRACKERS

Honorable mentions to this chapter include:
Fitbit
Apple Watch
Motiv Ring
WHOOP Strap
ECG monitors
Blood Pressure monitors
Pulse Oximeters

One more honorable mention, which is not a device but provides an essential service, is a website called www.mytavin.com. This site will alert you of nutrient deficiencies caused by pharmaceuticals. All you need to do is input the name of your prescription and you will get useful data. While all of this technology is exciting and fascinating, it's not meant to be used exclusively. Ideally, you can correlate the data collected with how you are feeling and learn more about your biology and what actions you can take according to these results to improve your health. As this technology continues to advance, we all must take charge of our health by, among other methods, testing and tracking.

One of the many problems with chronic diseases is that they not only progress slowly but consistently. The early symptoms, like inflammation, are often silent. Testing and tracking will allow you to learn about your health metrics and what is lurking deep inside of your body so you can make the appropriate adjustments early before the silent symptoms become noisy.

All chronic diseases begin with slight irregularities and then, over time, evolve into serious illnesses. Health issues such as high blood sugar, high blood pressure, nutrient deficiencies, unconscious stress (yes, there is such a thing—sometimes triggered by low-grade infections), and poor circulation can be subtle in the damage they are doing. If these are left unattended, they can advance and cause severe health problems.

It is a serious deficiency of our health-care system that millions of people can't afford these diagnostic tests. The prices of these tests are often highly inflated, and the costs vary according to insurance coverage, geographic location, and the type of test. Most insurance companies negotiate discounted rates with hospitals and labs. The result can be far less than the sticker price but can still be shockingly high.

I do not cover scans, MRIs, or X-rays, but if you need one of those, there are two sites that I found that may be helpful. Affordablescan. com and Clearhealthcosts.com can assist with obtaining the most affordable price on these tests.

I am sensitive to the fact that not everyone can afford these tests and devices. Perhaps, soon, there will be more competition to drive the prices down, making them more widely available and affordable. Having said that, I feel compelled to point out that regular tests have enormous benefits when part of one's preventive health plan. Certain conditions often begin without clear symptoms. Testing can evaluate one's health status and offer early detection, making conditions easier to treat. When early indications of underlying health issues are monitored, there is a greater likelihood of resolving the issue. Additionally, when one is taking certain medications, consistent blood work can identify if the dose is appropriate, if the intended goal is being accomplished, and even if medication-related side effects are occurring.

CAUTIONARY TALE

I recently heard a story about a woman who was feeling lethargic and had brain fog and loss of appetite. She consulted several doctors who concluded that the fact that her CBC blood test did not indicate infection meant that she was fine and simply experiencing age-related issues. After sleeping for twenty-nine hours straight and waking up with a swollen face, the woman was transported by ambulance to the hospital. A comprehensive metabolic panel revealed that she had stage four kidney disease and now was struggling to regain kidney function. Had this test been administered earlier, she may have had to spend a little more money upfront, but her kidney disease could have been identified and treated at a less serious stage.

ACTION STEPS

➢ Consider collecting your own quantitative data.

➢ Begin with basic blood work.

➢ Test for nutrient and mineral deficiencies.

➢ Determine the status of your gut microbiome by doing one of the many available tests.

➢ If you are trying to balance your hormones, and everyone should, do the DUTCH test.

➢ Consider an investment in the health-tracking devices discussed in this chapter. The main metrics to track are sleep, stress, movement, glucose, and heart rate.

CHAPTER 18

CLINICAL STUDIES:
It Is Best to Rely upon Evidence-Based Science and Medicine

CONFIRMATION BIAS AND THE ILLUSORY TRUTH EFFECT

Most people by nature are subject to confirmation bias. They search for and read only information that supports their previously held viewpoint, and they ignore or dispute anything contrary to their viewpoint. One of the problems with this is a concept called the "illusory truth effect." This is when we begin to believe something, anything, when it is repeated frequently, regardless of inherent validity. We confuse repetition with truth. This is a successful tool in both advertising and politics but not so with science.

SCIENTIFIC CONSENSUS

A loose explanation of the scientific method is that it begins with an observation or a hypothesis. This is followed by a theory that is established to explain the hypothesis or observation. Then, the theory is examined and tested to confirm its veracity. If the test of the theory eliminates enough uncertainty, it is a successful test, and the theory becomes a "proof of concept." At least one independent group must test this proof of concept for further validation and if this independent group finds the same results as the original researchers found for the proof of concept, the hypothesis becomes fact. The American news website Vox surveyed a group of scientific researchers and concluded that as careful as this process appears, there are plenty of problems. Some of the problems include the bias of peer reviews often due to professional jealousy, the relentless need of researchers to secure and sustain funding, and the publication of studies with faulty data because often flaws are undetected.[194]

> While the scientific method is not without inherent flaws and conflict, it does follow a specific structure to examine and prove facts and to avoid publishing false or invalidated data.

When considering clinical studies as a basis of fact and ultimate guidance, you are faced with the debate about "scientific consensus." While many rely upon scientific consensus, many others insist that it is a fallacy and is nonexistent. Scientific consensus is when many studies point to similar conclusions. The issue is when it becomes reflective of the popular opinion and not the basis of knowledge or evidence. Just because a big group of people believes something, doesn't necessarily make it true. Consensus has the propensity to be more aligned with probability than fact. While it can be a part of many ways to validate scientific claims, it should not be exclusively relied upon. There is a long list of consensus errors and inherent flaws. For one thing, scientific consensus changes over time. There are many other examples of this including the safety of smoking, sugar, margarine, and several previously approved pharmaceuticals. Personal values, bias, money, and conflicting motives are all factors that drive consensus but are unrelated to scientific evidence.

THE GOLD STANDARD?

I think this is worthy of discussion because there is a great deal of rigidity in science today and an immediate disregard for anything that isn't part of a large, randomized, double-blind, placebo-controlled clinical study. The designation "double-blind" indicates neither the participants nor the researchers know who receives the specific treatment. The goal of this is to prevent bias. While those are the "gold standard" of scientific research, these studies have inherent limitations. You must consider who is sponsoring any study as well as the profile of the participants. There are natural biases in the peer-review process toward accepting prevailing doctrines. Even the size of the study lends itself to problems. The gold standard emphasizes large studies, but often the effects diminish with larger studies and can't be replicated. There is a concept called the decline effect which describes the phenomenon that many results that are rigorously proven and accepted begin to fade in later studies. This is in part due to selective reporting. Scientists and scientific journals prefer positive data over studies that yield negative or no results. I think it would be useful if scientific journals published negative results. Studies can result in contradictory data when using different methodologies. As a result of the total reliance on this gold standard, debate and questioning are stymied. Instead of acknowledging that our biology is extraordinarily complex, and we simply don't know everything, we accept what scientific journals tell us to accept instead of constantly searching, investigating, and exploring new ideas and concepts.

THE VALUE OF OTHER STUDIES

Science does not encourage the questioning of facts that everyone has come to believe are true or the upsetting of the perceived order of things. Occasionally, it is not even facts but opinions that have been both presented and ultimately accepted as facts. As a result of this prevailing rigidity, observational studies, or epidemiological studies, are given little, if any, credence whatsoever. In fact, science considers observational studies to be the worst proof there is. Some say that you cannot know something to be true without confirming it with a randomized clinical study. While this could be true sometimes, it is simply not a universal truth. I am not suggesting that you seek your medical guidance exclusively from YouTube, I am suggesting that observational studies are not without merit. Observational studies usually rely upon personal testimony and can be flawed because people cannot be relied on to self-report accurately. They do, however, help with showing correlations between behaviors and outcomes. The results are subject to dispute because they are not conducted in a controlled test environment, and I am not suggesting that they should replace clinical studies, but they do provide value. Sometimes, conducting a randomized clinical study would be completely unnecessary because we can understand concepts from an observational perspective. An example of this is that we know when children play with matches, there is an increased rate of harm. There are no clinical studies to confirm this, but we know it to be true. In my opinion, the totality of the evidence should be considered.

COLLECTIVE EXPERIENCE

Another method that has not gained acceptance is "collective experience." This describes what biohackers do as they experiment relentlessly and share their results all over the world with other biohackers to indicate what is at least worth trying and what should not be tried. While it may not be prudent to rely completely on the results of collective experience, I strongly believe in reviewing and thinking about this method. We are all biochemically and genetically different, so what works well for one person may not work at all or even be harmful to another person. There is still value in others' experiences. Enough anecdotes can become empirical evidence.

HIERARCHY OF SCIENTIFIC EVIDENCE

Further confirmation that some of the currently accepted beliefs about science need to be updated is the "hierarchy of scientific evidence." At the top of this well-accepted pyramid of research is meta-analysis, which is the review of studies and the aggregation of the data. In an interesting article by Milton Packer, MD, titled "What Freddie Mercury Can Teach Us About Clinical Trials," he compares the approach of the totality of the evidence against meta-analysis. He asserts that these two concepts are the opposite of each other and maligns the very research tool which sits at the top of the hierarchy. He states, "A meta-analysis simply seeks to combine data in a thoughtless process that is uninformed by differences in trial methodology or patient populations. It yields a forced summary estimate that obscures meaning and truthfulness. In contrast, the 'totality of the evidence' approach is not a process of forced summation, but instead, it is an intellectually challenging process of reconciliation."[195]

CHIPS ON THE GOLD STANDARD

Recently, during the pandemic, two highly regarded scientific journals, *The Lancet* and *The New England Journal of Medicine*, published a story that contained incorrect information and had to retract the story. The panic and desperate need for actionable information were no doubt responsible for the uncharacteristic lack of vetting, but it just illustrated that nothing is without flaws. Another example of the potential problems with clinical studies is illustrated in the story about Yvelice Villaman-Bencosme, MD. This Florida doctor falsified clinical trial data in a study for an asthma drug for children. The justice system came down hard on this doctor, as it should have, and sentenced her to five years in prison.

One of the most egregious errors in science that I find stunning is that over fifty years ago, the sugar industry was able to bribe scientists from an Ivy League university to suppress evidence that processed sugars could cause heart disease and some cancers. This was right about the same time as scientists began demonizing fat, which has since been shown to be an essential part of our diet. As the study was revealing results that connected sucrose to serious health risks, the sugar industry abruptly shut the study down. While the sugar industry was and is aware of the confirmed link between sucrose and serious disease, they were able to successfully manipulate the research. There are similar examples of this involving tobacco research and the tobacco industry. I bring these up simply to exemplify the potential for clinical studies to be subject to fraud and manipulation. It is essential to learn who has sponsored a clinical study. Often the profit motive of the study sponsor impairs scientific integrity. It is not always easy to discern, but the conclusions of many studies are the result of data manipulation.

NUTRITIONAL STUDIES

Nutritional studies are the least dependable. Nutritional epidemiology is not the best method to rely on. It is dependent upon people self-reporting. People tend to self-report inaccurately about what they ate and how much of it they ate. Nutritional data lends itself to great manipulation to support any hypothesis. Even randomized controlled clinical studies are flawed because of the multitude of variables involved. Everyone's physiology and response are distinct, and foods interact with other foods often in an unanticipated way. Studies on food are not nearly as reliable as studies on drugs.

PREPRINTS

This is an emerging area of scientific publications. It describes medical manuscripts published for all to see before they have been peer reviewed. They represent an important method of open-source data sharing. Preprints are not without controversy. They are not always reliable due to a lack of being peer reviewed. There is little scientific quality control and potential for retraction. They do, however, become part of the scientific record and can assist in accelerating the scientific process. They cannot be relied upon with certainty but neither should they be ignored.

N OF 1

The single best, most dependable study is an N of 1. That is a sample size of one person, and you are that person. It is only through this endeavor that you can precisely determine what works best for your physiology and genetics.

Another aspect of clinical studies that requires change is the participant demographics. There is a serious health equity issue in that people of color and women are grossly underrepresented in clinical studies. While I am aware that not everyone has the time or inclination to do elaborate testing, the single most dependable study is an N of 1.

THE STORY OF MY SONS

My sons are three years apart in age, but when they were each five years old, I was advised by the school they were attending to consult a psychiatrist and medicate them for their "hyperactivity." The entire experience was truly horrifying and disappointing. At every turn, and there were countless turns, I was stunned by how the supposed "experts" had completely bought into the prevailing trend. The school administrators, teachers, and doctors spent exactly zero time pondering other solutions for young boys with excess energy. I suggested that the teachers send my boys outside to the playground to run laps when they could not sit still. And if you are thinking that the teachers can't allow the kids to be unsupervised, that was not an issue because I was forced to hire a "shadow" to monitor my boys' hyperactivity during the school day. While I won't go into my sincere feelings about the prevailing method of diagnosing ADHD (attention deficit hyperactivity disorder), I will discuss the absolutely appalling approach of prescribing hard-core prescription drugs for children.

Every doctor, and there were several, prescribed stimulant drugs for my young boys. For years, I refused to medicate my sons. Finally, when they turned thirteen years old, I agreed to a trial course of medication. I was concerned about the dosage because it occurred to me that children are rarely, if ever, included as participants in clinical trials. Drugs are usually tested on men. Women and children are not well represented in clinical studies. I appreciate that there are safety and ethical considerations about including children and women in clinical studies, but how is it that we gloss over administering the very same drugs without hesitation? Women and children are vastly different in both size and development than men. I questioned each doctor about the safety and efficacy of giving a dose of medication to a still-developing child that had only been tested on much larger, older men. I was consistently told, "this is how it's done." I was never able to quell my concerns about the unknown harmful side effects and ultimately stopped my kids from taking any more medication. The utter lack of evidence-based treatments for children is an issue that needs attention.

A compelling study that speaks to the scarce safety and efficacy data on medication for children is called "Clinical trials in children."[196] This study concludes that "the future health of children hinges on the success of pediatric trials."

ACTION STEPS

- ➢ Always do your due diligence when researching anything.

- ➢ Read several studies from different sources.

- ➢ Look for conclusions that can be repeated and not simple "one-offs."

- ➢ Never stop questioning. Ask, is there anything that could refute this?

- ➢ Try to determine who is the paid sponsor of a study and who owns the medical journals.

- ➢ Make every effort to distinguish marketing from science. This is not an easy task but a critical one.

CHAPTER 19

RESOURCES

I HAVE NO AFFILIATION WHATSOEVER with any of the following goods and services. These are listed simply as a reference tool and to be helpful. I have no profit motive and no conflict of interest in any of these resources. I urge everyone to do additional research before choosing any of the following.

CHAPTER 1: YOUR ORAL MICROBIOME

Toothpaste Brands

Davids Natural Toothpaste
Lumineux
Nature's Gate
Redmond Earthpaste Amazingly Natural Toothpaste
Dr. Brite
Zion Health
Dr. Bronner's All-One Toothpaste
Desert Essence
Hello
Primal Life Organics Toothpowder

Boka Ela Mint Toothpaste
Kopari Coconut Toothpaste
Weleda Plant-Rich Toothpaste
Schmidt's Wondermint Toothpaste

Mouthwash Brands

The Dirt Oil Pulling Mouthwash
Garner's Garden 100% All-Natural Mouthwash
Hello
Aesop
OLAS Marine Bio-Active Mouthrinse
Dr. Ginger's Coconut Oil Mouthwash
Auromere Ayurvedic Mouthwash
Desert Essence
Dr. Brite
Banyan Botanicals Daily Swish
Georganics
Lumineux

Dental Floss

Cocofloss
Hello
Public Goods
Dental Lace
RADIUS Natural Silk Floss
Boka Ela Minto Floss
Vömel
Desert Essence Tea Tree Oil Dental Floss
DrTung's Smart Floss
Eco-DenT GentleFloss

CHAPTER 4: STRESS

Meditation Apps

Headspace
Aura
Calm
Insight Timer
Sattva
Glo
Ensō
INSCAPE
iBreathe
Breethe
Oak
Waking Up
Buddhify
Unplug
Simple Habit
Ten Percent Happier

Stress-Monitoring Devices

Ōura Ring
Muse
Hapbee
WHOOP
Garmin
Samsung Galaxy Watch
Apple Watch
Fitbit
Google Wear OS smartwatch
Cove
Spire Stone
Flowtime
PIP

CHAPTER 5: TOXINS

Important Websites

Environmental Working Group (EWG.org)
Environmental Protections Agency (EPA.gov)
AirNow.gov
Lung.org
Pesticide Action Network (PANNA.org)

Most Contaminated Fish

Shark
Marlin
Swordfish
Lamprey
Pike
Tuna
Eel
Farmed fish
King mackerel
Opah

Safest Fish To Eat

Sardines
Herring
Cod
Alaskan salmon (wild-caught)

Nasa Air-Filtering Plants

Dwarf date palm
Areca palm
Boston fern

Kimberly Queen fern
English ivy
Lilyturf
Spider plant
Devil's ivy
Peace lily
Chinese evergreen
Bamboo palm
Broadleaf lady palm
Snake plant
Philodendron
Dracaena
Ficus benjamina
Rubber plant
Gerbera daisy
Dendrobium orchids
Phalaenopsis

Air Purifier Brands

Blueair
Honeywell
Coway
GermGuardian
Winix

Low-Toxin Or Toxin-Free Wine

Dry Farm Wines
SmartVine
Frey vineyards
Scout & Cellar
Inkarri

Low-Toxin Or Toxin-Free Beer

Wolaver's
Samuel Smith
Pinkus
Peak Brewing
Butte Creek Organic
Dogfish Head
Amarcord Brewery
Green's
Bison Brew

Certifications To Look For

USDA Organic Wine Certification
Demeter Biodynamic Certification
DetoxProject.org Glyphosate Residue Free Certification

Nontoxic Cookware Brands

Caraway
Our Place
Cuisinart
GreenPan
All-Clad Stainless Steel
Le Creuset
Xtrema Traditions
Green Earth
ZWILLING
Blue Diamond

Nontoxic Cleaning Product Brands

Branch Basics
Pure Haven

Greenshield Organic
Thrive Market
Meliora
Molly's Suds
Young Living
Dr. Bronner's
ECOS

Personal Care Product Brands

True Botanicals
Crunchi
Marie Veronique
Annmarie Gianni
Neal's Yard Remedies
Pure Haven

Other Sources To Consult

ECHA (European Chemicals Agency)
Think Dirty app
Whatsonmyfood.org

CHAPTER 6: SLEEP

Mattresses

Saatva
Avocado Green
Birch Natural Mattress
Awara Mattress
EcoCloud
Spindle Natural Latex Mattress
Amerisleep Organica

GhostBed Natural
My Green Mattress
Under the Canopy Hybrid Organic Latex Mattress
Happsy
Naturepedic
Zenhaven (Saatva)
Loom & Leaf (Saatva)
Brentwood Home
PlushBeds
Nest Bedding
Eco Terra
Essentia Mattress
Tuft & Needle
DreamCloud
Zoma
Natural Escape (My Green Mattress)
Helix

Blue-Light–Blocking Glasses

Gamma Ray
Felix Gray
Warby Parker
Cyxus
GUNNAR Intercept
Zenni Optical Blokz
TIJN
Privé Revaux
J+S Vision computer glasses
4EST Shades
COVRY
Baxter Blue Glasses
Livhò

MAXJULI
BLUblox

Light Boxes And Light Therapy

Carex Day-Light Classic Plus
Omnilux
Verilux
TheraLite
Circadian Optics
Aura Daylight Therapy Lamp (TheraLite)
Miroco
Philips
Alaska Northern Lights

CHAPTER 7: NUTRITION

Olive Oil

Kosterina
Laconiko
Bariani
Corto
Cobram Estate
California Olive Ranch
McEvoy Ranch
Olea Estates
Ottavio
Chaffin Family Orchards
Burroughs Family Farms

Fish

Wild Alaskan Company
Wild Planet Foods
Catch Sitka Seafood
Sea to Table
Vital Choice
Nordic Catch

Beef

ButcherBox
Grass Roots Farmers' CooperativeCrowd Cow
Perdue Farms
Silver Fern Farms
Chaffin Family Orchards
US Wellness Meats

Poultry

Porter Road
Cooks Venture
Crowd Cow
FarmFoods
FreshDirect
Murray's Chicken
ButcherBox

Labels To Look For

Certified Humane Raised & Handled
Animal Welfare Certified
Animal Welfare Approved

CHAPTER 9: RESPIRATORY PHYSIOLOGY

Mouth Tape

SomniFix

3M Micropore surgical tape

Other Resources

SOMA Breath online

Breatheology

Apps

iBreathe

Respira

Breathwrk

Wim Hof Method

The Breathing App

MindShift CBT

Breath Ball

Health through Breath

Kardia

Breathe2Relax

Just Relax

Steady-Breathing Meditation for Stress & Anxiety

Breathing-Mentor (This one is the focus of clinical study, "A Biofeedback App to Instruct Abdominal Breathing (Breathing-Mentor): Pilot Experiment" by Corinna Faust-Christmann et al.)

CHAPTER 12: LIGHT OPTIMIZATION

Light Bulbs

Incandescent
Halogen
LowBlueLights
Chromalux
GE
Satco
Philips
Lumiram
SYLVANIA

Photobiomodulation Red Light Therapy Devices

Joovv
Novaa Lab
PlatinumLED
MitoMIN
Beurer Infrared Heat Lamp
SGROW 45W Red Light
Red Light Man
Red Therapy Company

CHAPTER 13: HYDRATION

Water Filtration Systems

Reverse Osmosis Whole House System (the most effective type).
Aquasana
SpringWell Whole House Filter System
Pelican Water

Naturally Filtered
Crystal Quest
Home Master

Drinking Water Filters

Everpure
GE Dual Flow Water Filtration System
Whirlpool Water Purifier Filtration System
Berkey
Watts Premier
Brita
Soma
PUR
Waterdrop
Aquagear

Hydration Apps

Daily Water Tracker Reminder
Hydro Coach
WaterMinder
Water Drink Reminder
AQUALERT: Water Tracker Daily
My Water—Daily Hydration Tracker & Reminder
Drink Water Reminder N Tracker
Water Time Tracker & Drink Reminder
Plant Nanny
iHydrate
Water Your Body

CHAPTER 14: FASTING

Biosense (Breath Ketone Monitor & Mobile App)

Intermittent Fasting Apps

Window
InFasting
Fastic
Zero
Fastient
BodyFast
Vora
FastHabit
LIFE Fasting Tracker
DoFasting
MyFast

CHAPTER 15: SUPPLEMENTS

Best Brands

Designs for Health
Metagenics
Ortho Molecular Products
Pure Encapsulations
Thorne Research
Integrative Therapeutics
Standard Process
Apex Energetics
Douglas Labs
Klaire Labs
NOW Foods

Certifications

GMP (Good Manufacturing Practice)
QAI (Quality Assurance International)
USDA Organic

CHAPTER 16: GENETICS, EPIGENETICS, AND GENOMICS

Epigenetic Testing

Chronomics
Zymo Research
Muhdo
myDNAge
TruMeTruAge Explorer
Elysium Health Index Kit
TruDiagnostic
EpiAging USA

Genetic Testing

Preventive Genomics Clinic at Brigham Health/Brigham and Women's Hospital
Veritas Genetics
Dante Labs
CENTOGENE
Nebula Genomics
Toolbox Genomics
The DNA Company

CHAPTER 17: TESTING AND TRACKING

Labs For Blood Work

AMERICAN METABOLIC LABORATORIES
Labcorp
Quest Diagnostics

Private Md Labs

AmeriPath, Inc.
BioReference Laboratories, Inc.
GeneDx
Invitae Corporation
Millennium Health, LLC
Vibrant America
Advanced Diagnostic Laboratories
Cambridge Biomedical/BioAgilytix Boston
ZRT Laboratory

Direct-To-Consumer Blood Work

www.meenta.io (marketplace of testing products and laboratory services)
HealthCheckUSA
Life Extension
InsideTracker
Healthtestingcenters.com
Everlywell
Ulta Lab Tests
Walk-In Lab
HealthLabs
Request A Test
Let'sGetChecked

Testing Devices

Ōura Ring
Lumen

Continuous Glucose Monitors

Dexcom
Freestyle Libre
Eversense
Guardian Connect system
Care Touch
LEVELS

Hrv Monitors

Garmin
Fitbit
RENPHO
WHOOP

Smart Scales

Garmin
1byone
Nokia/Withings
FitTrack
Eufy
Fitbit
Under Armour
Weight Gurus
iHealth Core
Yunmai
RENPHO
Wyze Scale

Reference Websites

Mytavin.com (website lists nutrient deficiencies caused by medications)

ENDNOTES

1 Donna Shalala, CDA, n.d. https://www.cda.org/.

2 Tim Newman, "Causes and Treatment of Gingivitis," Medical News Today, January 5, 2018, https://www.medicalnewstoday.com/articles/241721#_noHeaderPrefixedContent.

3 "Biofilm," Lexico, https://www.lexico.com/en/definition/biofilm.

4 P. M. Preshaw, A. L. Alba, D. Herrera, S. Jepsen, A. Konstantinidis, K. Makrilakis, R. Taylor. "Periodontitis and Diabetes: A Two-Way Relationship." Diabetologia. Springer-Verlag, January 2012. https://www.ncbi.nlm.nih.gov/pmc/articles/PMC3228943/.

5 Priya Nimish Deo and Revati Deshmukh. "Oral Microbiome: Unveiling the Fundamentals." Journal of oral and maxillofacial pathology: JOMFP. Wolters Kluwer - Medknow, 2019. https://www.ncbi.nlm.nih.gov/pmc/articles/PMC6503789/.

6 "Periodontal Disease." Centers for Disease Control and Prevention. Centers for Disease Control and Prevention, July 10, 2013. https://www.cdc.gov/oralhealth/conditions/periodontal-disease.html.

7 Paul I. Eke, Wenche S. Borgnakke, Robert J. Genco. "Recent Epidemiologic Trends in Periodontitis in the USA." *Periodontology 2000* 82, no. 1 (2019): 257–67. https://doi.org/10.1111/prd.12323.

8 Walter J. Loesche. "Microbiology of Dental Decay and Periodontal Disease." Medical Microbiology. 4th edition. U.S. National Library of Medicine, January 1, 1996. https://www.ncbi.nlm.nih.gov/books/NBK8259/.

9 Walter J. Loesche. "Role of Streptococcus Mutans in Human Dental Decay." *Microbiological Reviews* 50, no. 4 (1986): 353–80. https://doi.org/10.1128/mr.50.4.353-380.1986.

10 "Dental Amalgam and Mercury by Birgit Calhoun (Amalgam Debate Forum) 8/30/2005 104341." CureZone.org: Educating Instead of Medicating, n.d. https://www.curezone.org/forums/fm.asp?i=104341.

11 Hector Jirau-Colón, Leonardo González-Parrilla, Jorge Martinez-Jiménez, Waldemar Adam, and Braulio Jiménez-Velez. "Rethinking the Dental Amalgam Dilemma: An Integrated Toxicological Approach." International journal of environmental research and public health. MDPI, March 22, 2019. https://www.ncbi.nlm.nih.gov/pmc/articles/PMC6466133/.

12 Mark C. Houston. "The Role of Mercury in Cardiovascular Disease." *Journal of Cardiovascular Diseases & Diagnosis* 02, no. 05 (2014). https://doi.org/10.4172/2329-9517.1000170.

13 Maria Messing, Letícia Chaves de Souza, Franco Cavalla, Krishna Kookal, Gabreilla Rizzo, Muhammad Walji, Renato Silva, and Ariadne Letra. "Investigating Potential Correlations between Endodontic Pathology and Cardiovascular Diseases Using Epidemiological and Genetic Approaches." Journal of Endodontics. Elsevier, January 17, 2019. https://www.sciencedirect.com/science/article/pii/S0099239918307489.

14 Y. W. Han, X. Wang. Mobile Microbiome: Oral Bacteria in Extra-Oral Infections and Inflammation." Journal of dental research. U.S. National Library of Medicine, n.d. https://pubmed.ncbi.nlm.nih.gov/23625375/.

15 Rizwan Ullah, Muhammed Sohail Zafar, and Nazish Shahani. "Potential Fluoride Toxicity from Oral Medicaments: A Review." Iranian journal of basic medical sciences. U.S. National Library of Medicine, n.d. https://pubmed.ncbi.nlm.nih.gov/29085574/.

16 Chia-Shu Lin. "Revisiting the Link between Cognitive Decline and Masticatory Dysfunction." BMC geriatrics. U.S. National Library of Medicine, n.d. https://pubmed.ncbi.nlm.nih.gov/29304748/.

    Akio Tada and Hiroko Miura. "Association between Mastication and Cognitive Status: A Systematic Review." *Archives of Gerontology and Geriatrics* 70 (2017): 44–53. https://doi.org/10.1016/j.archger.2016.12.006.

17 Debora Mackenzie. "We May Finally Know What Causes Alzheimer's – and How to Stop It." New Scientist, n.d. https://

www.newscientist.com/article/2191814-we-may-finally-
know-what-causes-alzheimers-and-how-to-stop-it/.

18   Stephen S. Dominy, C. Lynch, F. Ermini, M. Benedyk, A. Marczyk
     A, A. Konradi, M. Nguyen, U. Haditsch, D. Raha, C. Griffin, L.
     J. Holsinger, S. Arastu-Kapur, S. Kaba, A. Lee, M. I. Ryder, B.
     Potempa, P. Mydel, A. Hellvard, K. Adamowicz, H. Hasturk, G. D.
     Walker, E. C. Reynolds, R. L. M. Faull, M. A. Curtis, M. Dragunow,
     and Potempa. "Porphyromonas Gingivalis in Alzheimer's Disease
     Brains: Evidence for Disease Causation and Treatment with Small-
     Molecule Inhibitors." Science advances. U.S. National Library of
     Medicine, n.d. https://pubmed.ncbi.nlm.nih.gov/30746447/.

19   Rich Haridy. "How Mouthwash Can Alter Your Oral
     Microbiome and Potentially Damage Teeth." New Atlas,
     March 25, 2020. https://newatlas.com/health-wellbeing/
     common-mouthwash-saliva-acidic-alter-oral-microbiome/.

20   "Mapping the Motor Cortex." IGS RSS, n.d.
     https://hmpdACC.ORG/HMP.

21   Natren, Inc. "Battling Bad Bacteria." Natren, Inc., n.d. https://
     www.natren.com/blogs/news/battling-bad-bacteria/.

22   Ji Youn Yoo, Maureen Groer, Samia Valeria Ozorio Dutra, Anujit
     Sarkar, and Daniel Ian McSkimming. "Gut Microbiota and Immune
     System Interactions." Microorganisms. U.S. National Library of
     Medicine, n.d. https://pubmed.ncbi.nlm.nih.gov/33076307/.

23   Dorian McGavern. "The Gut Trains the Immune System to Protect
     the Brain." National Institute of Neurological Disorders and Stroke.
     U.S. Department of Health and Human Services, November 4, 2020.
     https://www.ninds.nih.gov/News-Events/News-and-Press-Releases/
     Press-Releases/gut-trains-immune-system-protect-brain.

24   Justin Sonnenberg. "Hunter-Gatherers of Tanzania Experience
     Seasonal Variation in Gut-Microbe Diversity." News Center, August
     24, 2017. https://med.stanford.edu/news/all-news/2017/08/
     hunter-gatherers-seasonal-gut-microbe-diversity-loss.html.

25   "Structure, Function and Diversity of the Healthy
     Human Microbiome." Nature 486, no. 7402 (2012):
     207–14. https://doi.org/10.1038/nature11234.

26 Top of Form Hale, W. G., Venetia A. Saunders, J.
P. Margham, and W. G. Hale. 2005. *Collins dictio-
nary of biology*. London: Collins.Bottom of Form

27 Juliana Durack, Susan V., and Lynch. "The Gut Microbiome:
Relationships with Disease and Opportunities for Therapy."
The Journal of experimental medicine. U.S. National Library of
Medicine, n.d. https://pubmed.ncbi.nlm.nih.gov/30322864/.

28 Anne Gnauck, Roger G. Lentle, Marlena C. Kruger. "The
Characteristics and Function of Bacterial Lipopolysaccharides
and Their Endotoxic Potential in Humans." International
reviews of immunology. U.S. National Library of Medicine,
n.d. https://pubmed.ncbi.nlm.nih.gov/26606737/.

29 Marie S. A. Palmnäs, T. E. Cowan, M. R. Bomhof, J. Su, R. A. Reimer,
H. J. Vogel, D. S. Hittel, and J. Shearer. "Low-Dose Aspartame
Consumption Differentially Affects Gut Microbiota-Host Metabolic
Interactions in the Diet-Induced Obese Rat." PloS one. U.S. National
Library of Medicine, n.d. https://pubmed.ncbi.nlm.nih.gov/25313461/.

30 J. Phillip Karl, A. M. Hatch, S. M. Arcidiacono, S. C. Pearce, I.
G. Pantoja-Feliciano, L. A> Doherty, J. W. Soares. "Effects of
Psychological, Environmental and Physical Stressors on the Gut
Microbiota." Frontiers in microbiology. U.S. National Library of
Medicine, n.d. https://pubmed.ncbi.nlm.nih.gov/30258412/.

31 Lucy J. Mailing, J. M. Allen, T. W. Buford, C. J. Fields, and J. A.
Woods. "Exercise and the Gut Microbiome: A Review of the
Evidence, Potential Mechanisms, and Implications for Human
Health." Exercise and sport sciences reviews. U.S. National Library
of Medicine, n.d. https://pubmed.ncbi.nlm.nih.gov/30883471/.

32 Samantha R. Ellis, Mimi Nguyen, Alexandra R. Vaughn, Manisha
Notay, Waqas A. Burney, Simran Sandhu, and Raja K. Sivamani.
"The Skin and Gut Microbiome and Its Role in Common
Dermatologic Conditions." Microorganisms. MDPI, November 11,
2019. http://www.ncbi.nlm.nih.gov/pmc/articles/PMC6920876.

33 Whitney P. Bowe and Alan C. Logan. "Acne Vulgaris, Probiotics
and the Gut-Brain-Skin Axis - Back to the Future?" *Gut Pathogens*
3, no. 1 (2011): 1. https://doi.org/10.1186/1757-4749-3-1.

34 Ashley Yeager, The Scientist March 4. "Can the Flu and Other
    Viruses Cause Neurodegeneration?" RealClearScience, n.d.
    https://www.realclearscience.com/2019/03/04/can_the_flu_
    and_other_viruses_cause_neurodegeneration_284984.html.

35 Michela Deleidi and Ole Isacson. "Viral and Inflammatory
    Triggers of Neurodegenerative Diseases." Science transla-
    tional medicine. U.S. National Library of Medicine, n.d.
    https://www.ncbi.nlm.nih.gov/pmc/articles/3982831/.

36 Firdaus S. Dhabhar. "Effects of Stress on Immune Function:
    The Good, the Bad, and the Beautiful." Immunologic
    research. U.S. National Library of Medicine, n.d.
    https://pubmed.ncbi.nlm.nih.gov/24798553/.

37 Suzanne C. Segerstrom and Gregory E. Miller. "Psychological
    Stress and the Human Immune System: A Meta-Analytic Study of
    30 Years of Inquiry." Psychological bulletin. U.S. National Library
    of Medicine, n.d. https://pubmed.ncbi.nlm.nih.gov/15250815/.

38 Anitra C. Carr and Silvia Maggini. "Vitamin C and Immune
    Function." Nutrients. U.S. National Library of Medicine,
    n.d. https://pubmed.ncbi.nlm.nih.gov/29099763/.

39 Cynthia Aranow. "Vitamin D and the Immune System." Journal of
    investigative medicine : the official publication of the American
    Federation for Clinical Research. U.S. National Library of
    Medicine, n.d. https://pubmed.ncbi.nlm.nih.gov/21527855/.

40 Peter R. Hoffman and Marla J. Berry. "The Influence
    of Selenium on Immune Responses." Molecular nutri-
    tion & food research. U.S. National Library of Medicine,
    n.d. https://pubmed.ncbi.nlm.nih.gov/18384097/.

41 Mei-Chun Kuo, M. J., C. Y. Weng, C. L. Ha, and Wu. "Ganoderma
    Lucidum Mycelia Enhance Innate Immunity by Activating
    NF-Kappab." Journal of ethnopharmacology. U.S. National Library
    of Medicine, n.d. https://pubmed.ncbi.nlm.nih.gov/16169168/.

42 Antonio Carrillo-Vico, Patricia Lardone, Nuria Álvarez-Sánchez,
    Ana Rodríguez-Rodríguez, and Juan Guerrero. "Melatonin: Buffering
    the Immune System." International Journal of Molecular Sciences
    14, no. 4 (2013): 8638–83. https://doi.org/10.3390/ijms14048638.

43 Tania Siqueiros-Cendón, Sigifredo Arévalo-Gallegos, Blanca
    Flor Iglesias-Figueroa, Isui Abril García-Montoya, José Salazar-
    Martínez, and Quintín Rascón-Cruz. "Immunomodulatory
    Effects of Lactoferrin." *Acta Pharmacologica Sinica* 35, no.
    5 (2014): 557–66. https://doi.org/10.1038/aps.2013.200.

44 Michael R. Hamblin. "Mechanisms and Applications of the Anti-
    Inflammatory Effects of Photobiomodulation." *AIMS Biophysics*
    4, no. 3 (2017): 337–61. https://doi.org/10.3934/biophy.2017.3.337.

45 Tiina Karu. "Is It Time to Consider Photobiomodulation as a
    Drug Equivalent?" *Photomedicine and Laser Surgery* 31, no.
    5 (2013): 189–91. https://doi.org/10.1089/pho.2013.3510.

46 Ann Liebert, Brian Bicknell, Wayne Markman, and Hosen Kiat.
    "A Potential Role for Photobiomodulation Therapy in Disease
    Treatment and Prevention in the Era of Covid-19." *Aging and dis-
    ease* 11, no. 6 (2020): 1352. https://doi.org/10.14336/ad.2020.0901.

47 A. Mooventhan and L. Nivethitha. Scientific Evidence-Based
    Effects of Hydrotherapy on Various Systems of the Body." North
    American journal of medical sciences. U.S. National Library of
    Medicine, n.d. https://pubmed.ncbi.nlm.nih.gov/24926444/.

48 C. Franceschi and J. Campisi. "Chronic Inflammation (Inflammaging)
    and Its Potential Contribution to Age-Associated Diseases." *The
    Journals of Gerontology Series A: Biological Sciences and Medical
    Sciences* 69, no. Suppl 1 (2014). https://doi.org/10.1093/gerona/glu057.

49 Wildmind Meditation News, "Can Training Soldiers
    to Meditate Combat PTSD?" Wildmind Meditation,
    May 3, 2010, https://www.wildmind.org/blogs/news/
    can-training-soldiers-to-meditate-combat-ptsd.

50 Daniel Schneider. "Mindfulness Helps Soldiers
    Cope." www.army.mil, n.d. https://www.army.mil/
    article/43269/mindfulness_helps_soldiers_cope.

51 "Harvard Unveils MRI Study Proving Meditation Literally
    Rebuilds the Brain's Gray Matter in 8 Weeks." FEELguide,
    November 19, 2014. https://www.feelguide.com/2014/11/19/
    harvard-unveils-mri-study-proving-meditation-literal-
    ly-rebuilds-the-brains-gray-matter-in-8-weeks/.

52 Mark Wheeler. "Forever Young: Meditation Might Slow the Age-Related Loss of Gray Matter in the Brain, Say UCLA Researchers." UCLA. UCLA, February 5, 2015. https://newsroom.ucla.edu/releases/forever-young-meditation-might-slow-the-age-related-loss-of-gray-matter-in-the-brain-say-ucla-researchers.

53 "Role and Efficacy of Positive Thinking on Stress...," n.d. https://www.researchgate.net/publication/321212701_Role_and_efficacy_of_Positive_Thinking_on_Stress_Management_and_Creative_Problem_Solving_for_Adolescents.

54 Mayo Clinic Staff. Positive Thinking: Stop Negative Self-Talk to Reduce Stress." Mayo Clinic. Mayo Foundation for Medical Education and Research, January 21, 2020. https://www.mayoclinic.org/healthy-lifestyle/stress-management/in-depth/positive-thinking/art-20043950.

55 Andrea Beetz, Kerstin Uvnäs-Moberg, Henri Julius, and Kurt Kotrschal. "Psychosocial and Psychophysiological Effects of Human-Animal Interactions: The Possible Role of Oxytocin." *Frontiers in Psychology* 3 (2012). https://doi.org/10.3389/fpsyg.2012.00234.

56 "Scientists Find Genetic Factor in Stress Response Variability." National Institute on Alcohol Abuse and Alcoholism. U.S. Department of Health and Human Services, n.d. https://www.niaaa.nih.gov/news-events/news-releases/scientists-find-genetic-factor-stress-response-variability.

57 Bettina Olsen. "Why Are Trace Chemicals Showing up in Umbilical Cord Blood?" Scientific American. Scientific American, September 1, 2012. https://www.scientificamerican.com/article/chemicals-umbilical-cord-blood/.

58 "Summary of the Toxic Substances Control Act." EPA. Environmental Protection Agency, n.d. https://www.epa.gov/laws-regulations/summary-toxic-substances-control-act.

59 Susan M. Duty, Narendra P. Singh, Manori J. Silva, Dana B. Barr, John W. Brock, Louise Ryan, Robert F. Herrick, David C. Christiani, and Russ Hauser. "The Relationship between Environmental Exposures to Phthalates and DNA Damage in Human Sperm Using the Neutral Comet Assay." *Environmental Health Perspectives* 111, no. 9 (2003): 1164–69. https://doi.org/10.1289/ehp.5756.

60 Russ Hauser, Susan Duty, Linda Godfrey-Bailey, and Antonia M. Calafat. "Medications as a Source of Human Exposure to Phthalates." *Environmental Health Perspectives* 112, no. 6 (2004): 751–53. https://doi.org/10.1289/ehp.6804.

61 Carl-Gustaf Bornehag, Jan Sundell, Charles J. Weschler, Torben Sigsgaard, Björn Lundgren, Mikael Hasselgren, and Linda Hägerhed-Engman. "The Association between Asthma and Allergic Symptoms in Children and Phthalates in House Dust: A Nested Case–Control Study." *Environmental Health Perspectives* 112, no. 14 (2004): 1393–97. https://doi.org/10.1289/ehp.7187.

62 "Phthalates: Are They Safe?" CBS News. CBS Interactive, n.d. https://www.cbsnews.com/news/phthalates-are-they-safe/.

63 Lisa M. Weatherly, Andrew J. Nelson, Juyoung Shim, Abigail M. Riitano, Erik D. Gerson, Andrew J. Hart, Jaime de Juan-Sanz, et al. "Antimicrobial Agent Triclosan Disrupts Mitochondrial Structure, Revealed by Super-Resolution Microscopy, and Inhibits Mast Cell Signaling via Calcium Modulation." *Toxicology and Applied Pharmacology* 349 (2018): 39–54. https://doi.org/10.1016/j.taap.2018.04.005.

64 Matej Skocaj, Metka Filipic, Jana Petkovic, and Sasa Novak. "Titanium Dioxide in Our Everyday Life; Is It Safe?" *Radiology and Oncology* 45, no. 4 (2011). https://doi.org/10.2478/v10019-011-0037-0.

65 TY - JOUR
      AU - Krüger, Kristin
      AU - Cossais, François
      AU - Neve, Horst.
      AU - Klempt, Martin
      PY - 2014/05/01
      SP -
      T1 - Titanium dioxide nanoparticles activate IL8-related inflammatory pathways in human colonic epithelial Caco-2 cells
      VL - 16
      DO - 10.1007/s11051-014-2402-6
      JO - Journal of Nanoparticle Research
      ER -

66 "Know Your Choices." EWG, January 20, 2021. http://www.ewg.org/.

67 Vijay Kumar and Kiran Dip Gill. "Aluminium Neurotoxicity: Neurobehavioural and Oxidative Aspects." *Archives of Toxicology* 83, no. 11 (2009): 965–78. https://doi.org/10.1007/s00204-009-0455-6.

68 Anne E. Nigra, K. E. Nachman, D. C. Love, M. Grau-Perez, and A. Navas-Acien. "Poultry Consumption and Arsenic Exposure in the U.S. Population." Environmental health perspectives. U.S. National Library of Medicine, n.d. https://pubmed.ncbi.nlm.nih.gov/27735790/.

69 D. Wilson. "Arsenic Consumption in the United States." Journal of environmental health. U.S. National Library of Medicine, n.d. https://pubmed.ncbi.nlm.nih.gov/26591332/.

70 Soile Tapio. "Arsenic in the Aetiology of Cancer." Mutation Research/ Reviews in Mutation Research, May 27, 2014. https://www.academia.edu/5863513/Arsenic_in_the_aetiology_of_cancer.

C. J. Chen., S. L. Wang, J. M. Chiou, C. H. Tseng, H. Y. Chiou, Y. M. Hsueh, S. Y. Chen, M. M. Wu, and M. S. Lai. "Arsenic and Diabetes and Hypertension in Human Populations: A Review." Toxicology and applied pharmacology. U.S. National Library of Medicine, n.d. https://pubmed.ncbi.nlm.nih.gov/17307211/.

71 Geir Bjørklund, Alexey A. Tinkov, Maryam Dadar, Md. Mostafizur Rahman, Salvatore Chirumbolo, Anatoly V. Skalny, Margarita G. Skalnaya, Boyd E. Haley, Olga P. Ajsuvakova, and Jan Aaseth. "Insights into the Potential Role of Mercury in Alzheimer's Disease." *Journal of Molecular Neuroscience*, 2019. https://doi.org/10.1007/s12031-019-01274-3.

72 Jong Suk Park, Kyoung Hwa Ha, Ka He, and Dae Jung Kim. "Association between Blood Mercury Level and Visceral Adiposity in Adults." *Diabetes & Metabolism Journal* 41, no. 2 (2017): 113. https://doi.org/10.4093/dmj.2017.41.2.113.

73 Diana Pisa, Ruth Alonso, Angeles Juarranz, Alberto Rábano, and Luis Carrasco. "Direct Visualization of Fungal Infection in Brains from Patients with Alzheimer's Disease." *Journal of Alzheimer's Disease* 43, no. 2 (2014): 613–24. https://doi.org/10.3233/jad-141386.

74 "The Proposition 65 List." Oehha.ca.gov, n.d. https://oehha.ca.gov/proposition-65/proposition-65-list.

75 "Popular Brands of Beer & Wine Found to
     Contain Glyphosate." USpirg.org

76 Erin Suni. "Sleep Statistics - Facts and Data about Sleep 2021."
     Sleep Foundation, November 2, 2021. https://www.sleep-
     foundation.org/how-sleep-works/sleep-facts-statistics.

77 "When You're Tired, Your Brain Cells Actually Slow Down."
     ScienceDaily. ScienceDaily, November 8, 2017. https://www.
     sciencedaily.com/releases/2017/11/171108124201.htm.

78 N. Asif N, R. Iqbal R, C. F. Nazir CF. "Human Immune System
     during Sleep." American journal of clinical and experi-
     mental immunology. U.S. National Library of Medicine,
     n.d. https://pubmed.ncbi.nlm.nih.gov/29348984/.

     Van Dongen, Hans P.A., Greg Maislin, Janet M. Mullington, and David
     F. Dinges. "The Cumulative Cost of Additional Wakefulness: Dose-
     Response Effects on Neurobehavioral Functions and Sleep Physiology
     from Chronic Sleep Restriction and Total Sleep Deprivation." Sleep
     26, no. 2 (2003): 117–26. https://doi.org/10.1093/sleep/26.2.117.

79 Ibid.

80 Katherine Harmon. Rare Genetic Mutation Lets Some
     People Function with Less Sleep." Scientific American.
     Scientific American, August 13, 2009. https://www.scientifi-
     camerican.com/article/genetic-mutation-sleep-less/.

81 T. Takumi, K. Taguchi, S. Miyake, et al. "A Light-Independent
     Oscillatory Gene mper3 in Mouse SCN and OVLT." The EMBO Journal
     17, no. 16 (1998): 4753–59. https://doi.org/10.1093/emboj/17.16.4753.

82 Lauren P. Shearman, Xiaowei Jin, Choogon Lee, Steven M.
     Reppert, and David R. Weaver. "Targeted Disruption of the
     mper3 Gene: Subtle Effects on Circadian Clock Function."
     Molecular and Cellular Biology 20, no. 17 (2000): 6269–75.
     https://doi.org/10.1128/mcb.20.17.6269-6275.2000.

83 Nadia Aalling Jessen, Anne Sofie Munk, Iben Lundgaard,
     and Maiken Nedergaard. "The Glymphatic System: A
     Beginner's Guide." Neurochemical Research 40, no. 12 (2015):
     2583–99. https://doi.org/10.1007/s11064-015-1581-6.

84 Karen R. Siegel, Kai McKeever Bullard, Giuseppina Imperatore, Henry S. Kahn, Aryeh D. Stein, Mohammed K. Ali, and K. M. Narayan. "Association of Higher Consumption of Foods Derived from Subsidized Commodities with Adverse Cardiometabolic Risk among US Adults." *JAMA Internal Medicine* 176, no. 8 (2016): 1124. https://doi.org/10.1001/jamainternmed.2016.2410.

85 Crystal Gammon. "Weed-Whacking Herbicide Proves Deadly to Human Cells." Scientific American. Scientific American, June 23, 2009. https://www.scientificamerican.com/article/weed-whacking-herbicide-p/.

86 Anthony Samsel and Stephanie Seneff. "Glyphosate, Pathways to Modern Diseases II: Celiac Sprue and Gluten Intolerance." *Interdisciplinary Toxicology* 6, no. 4 (2013): 159–84. https://doi.org/10.2478/intox-2013-0026.

87 "World Health Organization Labels Glyphosate Probable Carcinogen." Environmental Working Group, October 27, 2021. https://www.ewg.org/news-insights/news-release/world-health-organization-labels-glyphosate-probable-carcinogen.

88 Doris Cellarius. "Sierra Club Grassroots Network." Monsanto's sealed documents reveal truth behind Roundup's toxicological dangers | Grassroots Network, n.d. https://content.sierraclub.org/grassrootsnetwork/team-news/2015/09/monsanto-s-sealed-documents-reveal-truth-behind-roundup-s-toxicological-dangers.

89 Mohammad G. Saklayen. "The Global Epidemic of the Metabolic Syndrome." *Current Hypertension Reports* 20, no. 2 (2018). https://doi.org/10.1007/s11906-018-0812-z.

90 Marta Garaulet and Purificación Gómez-Abellán. "Timing of Food Intake and Obesity: A Novel Association." *Physiology & Behavior* 134 (2014): 44–50. https://doi.org/10.1016/j.physbeh.2014.01.001.

91 Stephen Anton and Christiaan Leeuwenburgh. "Fasting or Caloric Restriction for Healthy Aging." *Experimental Gerontology* 48, no. 10 (2013): 1003–5. https://doi.org/10.1016/j.exger.2013.04.011.

92 Jo Ann Carson, Alice H. Lichtenstein, Cheryl A.M. Anderson, Lawrence J. Appel, Penny M. Kris-Etherton, Katie A. Meyer, Kristina Petersen, Tamar Polonsky, and Linda Van Horn. "Dietary

Cholesterol and Cardiovascular Risk: A Science Advisory from the American Heart Association." *Circulation* 141, no. 3 (2020). https://doi.org/10.1161/cir.0000000000000743.

93 Richa Tulsian, Nikkhil Velingkaar, and Roman Kondratov. "Caloric Restriction Effects on Liver Mtor Signaling Are Time-of-Day Dependent." *Aging* 10, no. 7 (2018): 1640–48. https://doi.org/10.18632/aging.101498.

94 Anna E. Thalacker-Mercer, James C. Fleet, Bruce A. Craig, Nadine S. Carnell, and Wayne W. Campbell. "Inadequate Protein Intake Affects Skeletal Muscle Transcript Profiles in Older Humans." *The American Journal of Clinical Nutrition* 85, no. 5 (2007): 1344–52. https://doi.org/10.1093/ajcn/85.5.1344.

95 "65 Alternative Names of Sugar," The Health Sciences Academy, https://thehealthsciencesacademy.org/wp-content/uploads/2014/08/The-Health-Sciences-Academy_65-Names-Of-Sugar.pdf.

96 Chun-Yi Ng, Xin-Fang Leong, Norliana Masbah, Siti Khadijah Adam, Yusof Kamisah, and Kamsiah Jaarin. "Heated Vegetable Oils and Cardiovascular Disease Risk Factors." *Vascular Pharmacology* 61, no. 1 (2014): 1–9. https://doi.org/10.1016/j.vph.2014.02.004.

97 James J. DiNicolantonio and James H. O'Keefe. "Omega-6 Vegetable Oils as a Driver of Coronary Heart Disease: The Oxidized Linoleic Acid Hypothesis." *Open Heart* 5, no. 2 (2018). https://doi.org/10.1136/openhrt-2018-000898.

98 E. Patterson, R. Wall, G. F. Fitzgerald, R. P. Ross, and C. Stanton. "Health Implications of High Dietary Omega-6 Polyunsaturated Fatty Acids." *Journal of Nutrition and Metabolism* 2012 (2012): 1–16. https://doi.org/10.1155/2012/539426.

99 Núria Carranco, Mireia Farrés-Cebrián, Javier Saurina, and Oscar Núñez. "Authentication and Quantitation of Fraud in Extra Virgin Olive Oils Based on HPLC-UV Fingerprinting and Multivariate Calibration." *Foods* 7, no. 4 (2018): 44. https://doi.org/10.3390/foods7040044.

100 Peter Osborne, "Guidelines for Avoiding Gluten (Unsafe Ingredients for Gluten Sensitivity)" Gluten Free Society Blog, Accessed November 22, 2021, https://www.glutenfreesociety.org/guidelines-for-avoiding-gluten-unsafe-ingredients-for-gluten-sensitivity/.

101 "The Many Names of Monosodium Glutamate (MSG)" Fooducate, November 4, 2010, https://www.fooducate.com/community/post/The-Many-Names-of-Monosodium-Glutamate-MSG/57A333FD-2C35-9C9D-4EE7-B9C0CD3D6682.

102 Di Liegro CM, Schiera G, Proia P, Di Liegro I. Physical Activity and Brain Health. Genes (Basel). 2019 Sep 17;10(9):720. doi: 10.3390/genes10090720. PMID: 31533339; PMCID: PMC6770965.

103 Matthew S. Feigenbaum and Michael L. Pollock. "Prescription of Resistance Training for Health and Disease." *Medicine & Science in Sports & Exercise* 31, no. 1 (1999): 38–45. https://doi.org/10.1097/00005768-199901000-00008.

104 Trine Karlsen, Inger-Lise Aamot, Mark Haykowsky, and Øivind Rognmo. "High Intensity Interval Training for Maximizing Health Outcomes." *Progress in Cardiovascular Diseases* 60, no. 1 (2017): 67–77. https://doi.org/10.1016/j.pcad.2017.03.006.

105 Christian M. Werner, Anne Hecksteden, Arne Morsch, Joachim Zundler, Melissa Wegmann, Jürgen Kratzsch, Joachim Thiery, et al. "Differential Effects of Endurance, Interval, and Resistance Training on Telomerase Activity and Telomere Length in a Randomized, Controlled Study." *European Heart Journal* 40, no. 1 (2018): 34–46. https://doi.org/10.1093/eurheartj/ehy585.

106 Mikael Flockhart, Lina C. Nilsson, Senna Tais, Björn Ekblom, William Apró, and Filip J. Larsen. "Excessive Exercise Training Causes Mitochondrial Functional Impairment and Decreases Glucose Tolerance in Healthy Volunteers." *Cell Metabolism* 33, no. 5 (2021). https://doi.org/10.1016/j.cmet.2021.02.017.

107 John D. Akins, Charles K. Crawford, Heath M. Burton, Anthony S. Wolfe, Emre Vardarli, and Edward F. Coyle. "Inactivity Induces Resistance to the Metabolic Benefits Following Acute Exercise." *Journal of Applied Physiology* 126, no. 4 (2019): 1088–94. https://doi.org/10.1152/japplphysiol.00968.2018.

108 Kévin Contrepois, Si Wu, Kegan J. Moneghetti, Daniel Hornburg, Sara Ahadi, Ming-Shian Tsai, Ahmed A. Metwally, et al. "Molecular Choreography of Acute Exercise." *Cell* 181, no. 5 (2020). https://doi.org/10.1016/j.cell.2020.04.043.

109 Brian Kern, MD. "Hyperventilation Syndrome." Practice Essentials, Pathophysiology, Etiology. Medscape, October 16, 2021. https:// emedicine.medscape.com/article/807277-overview.

110 M. N. Alshak, M. Das J. "Neuroanatomy, Sympathetic Nervous System." National Center for Biotechnology Information. U.S. National Library of Medicine, n.d. https://pubmed.ncbi.nlm.nih.gov/31194352/.

111 Otto Muzik, Kaice T. Reilly, and Vaibhav A. Diwadkar. "'Brain over Body'–A Study on the Willful Regulation of Autonomic Function during Cold Exposure." *NeuroImage* 172 (2018): 632–41. https://doi.org/10.1016/j.neuroimage.2018.01.067.

112 Peng Li, Wiktor A. Janczewski, Kevin Yackle, Kaiwen Kam, Silvia Pagliardini, Mark A. Krasnow, and Jack L. Feldman. "The Peptidergic Control Circuit for Sighing." *Nature* 530, no. 7590 (2016): 293–97. https://doi.org/10.1038/nature16964.

113 Elke Vlemincx, Ilse Van Diest, and Omer Van den Bergh. "A Sigh of Relief or a Sigh to Relieve: The Psychological and Physiological Relief Effect of Deep Breaths." *Physiology & Behavior* 165 (2016): 127–35. https://doi.org/10.1016/j.physbeh.2016.07.004.

114 Tavia Gordon. "Menopause and Coronary Heart Disease." *Annals of Internal Medicine* 89, no. 2 (1978): 157. https://doi.org/10.7326/0003-4819-89-2-157.

115 Hisham Mohammed, I. Alasdair Russell, Rory Stark, Oscar M. Rueda, Theresa E. Hickey, Gerard A. Tarulli, Aurelien A. Serandour, et al. "Progesterone Receptor Modulates ERA Action in Breast Cancer." *Nature* 523, no. 7560 (2015): 313–17. https://doi.org/10.1038/ nature14583. Jason S. Carroll, Theresa E. Hickey, Gerard A. Tarulli, Michael Williams, and Wayne D. Tilley. "Deciphering the Divergent Roles of Progestogens in Breast Cancer." *Nature Reviews Cancer* 17, no. 1 (2016): 54–64. https://doi.org/10.1038/nrc.2016.116.

116 Arthur Hartz, Tao He, and John Jacob Ross. "Risk Factors for Colon Cancer in 150,912 Postmenopausal Women." *Cancer Causes & Control* 23, no. 10 (2012): 1599–1605. https://doi.org/10.1007/s10552-012-0037-4.

117 Thomas G. Travison, Andre B. Araujo, Amy B. O'Donnell, Varant Kupelian, and John B. McKinlay. "A Population-Level Decline in Serum Testosterone Levels in American Men."

The Journal of Clinical Endocrinology & Metabolism 92, no. 1 (2007): 196–202. https://doi.org/10.1210/jc.2006-1375.

118 M. Maggio, Basaria S., Ceda G. P., Ble A., Ling S. M., Bandinelli S., Valenti G., and Ferrucci L. "The Relationship between Testosterone and Molecular Markers of Inflammation in Older Men." Journal of endocrinological investigation. U.S. National Library of Medicine, n.d. https://pubmed.ncbi.nlm.nih.gov/16760639/.

119 Carlo Pergola, Anja Rogge, Gabriele Dodt, Hinnak Northoff, Christina Weinigel, Dagmar Barz, Olof Rådmark, Lidia Sautebin, and Oliver Werz. "Testosterone Suppresses Phospholipase D, Causing Sex Differences in Leukotriene Biosynthesis in Human Monocytes." *The FASEB Journal* 25, no. 10 (2011): 3377–87. https://doi.org/10.1096/fj.11-182758.

120 Susan R. Davis, R. Baber, N. Panay, J. Bitzer, S. C. Perez, R. M. Islam, A. M. Kaunitz, S. A. Kingsberg, I. Lambrinoudaki, J. Liu, S. J. Parish, J. Pinkerton, J. Rymer, J. A. Simon, L. Vignozzi, and M. E. Wierman. "Global Consensus Position Statement on the Use of Testosterone Therapy for Women." The Journal of clinical endocrinology and metabolism. U.S. National Library of Medicine, n.d. https://pubmed.ncbi.nlm.nih.gov/31498871/.

121 Sanjay K. Agarwal, AnnaMarie Daniels, Steven R. Drosman, Laurence Udoff, Warren G. Foster, Malcolm C. Pike, Darcy V. Spicer, and John R. Daniels. "Treatment of Endometriosis with the GNRHA Deslorelin and Add-Back Estradiol and Supplementary Testosterone." *BioMed Research International* 2015 (2015): 1–9. https://doi.org/10.1155/2015/934164.

122 Hillary D. White and Thomas D. Robinson. "A Novel Use for Testosterone to Treat Central Sensitization of Chronic Pain in Fibromyalgia Patients." *International Immunopharmacology* 27, no. 2 (2015): 244–48. https://doi.org/10.1016/j.intimp.2015.05.020.

123 H. Wang, W. Olivero, D. Wang, and G. Lanzino. "Cold as a Therapeutic Agent." *Acta Neurochirurgica* 148, no. 5 (2006): 565–70. https://doi.org/10.1007/s00701-006-0747-z.

Masayuki Saito. "Human Brown Adipose Tissue: Regulation and Anti-Obesity Potential." Endocrine Journal. The Japan

Endocrine Society, May 31, 2014. https://www.jstage.jst.
go.jp/article/endocrj/61/5/61_EJ13-0527/_article.

124 Nikolai A. Shevchuk. "Adapted Cold Shower as a Potential
Treatment for Depression." *Medical Hypotheses* 70, no. 5 (2008):
995–1001. https://doi.org/10.1016/j.mehy.2007.04.052.

125 Tiina M. Mäkinen, Matti Mäntysaari, Tiina Pääkkönen, Jari
Jokelainen, Lawrence A. Palinkas, Juhani Hassi, Juhani Leppäluoto,
Kari Tahvanainen, and Hannu Rintamäki. "Autonomic Nervous
Function during Whole-Body Cold Exposure before and after Cold
Acclimation." *Aviation, Space, and Environmental Medicine* 79,
no. 9 (2008): 875–82. https://doi.org/10.3357/asem.2235.2008.

126 L. Janský, D. Pospíšilová, S. Honzová, B. Uličný, P. Šrámek,
V. Zeman, and J. Kamínková. "Immune System of Cold-
Exposed and Cold-Adapted Humans." *European Journal of
Applied Physiology and Occupational Physiology* 72-72, no.
5-6 (1996): 445–50. https://doi.org/10.1007/bf00242274.

127 A. A. van der Lans, Joris Hoeks, Boudewijn Brans, Guy H.E.J.
Vijgen, Mariëlle G.W. Visser, Maarten J. Vosselman, Jan Hansen,
et al. "Cold Acclimation Recruits Human Brown Fat and Increases
Nonshivering Thermogenesis." *Journal of Clinical Investigation*
123, no. 8 (2013): 3395–3403. https://doi.org/10.1172/jci68993.

128 Saito, Masayuki. "Human Brown Adipose Tissue: Regulation
and Anti-Obesity Potential." *Endocrine Journal* 61, no. 5
(2014): 409–16. https://doi.org/10.1507/endocrj.ej13-0527.

129 Barbara Cannon and Jan Nedergaard. "Brown Adipose Tissue:
Function and Physiological Significance." *Physiological Reviews* 84,
no. 1 (2004): 277–359. https://doi.org/10.1152/physrev.00015.2003.

130 Barbara Cannon and Jan Nedergaard. "Nonshivering
Thermogenesis and Its Adequate Measurement in
Metabolic Studies." *Journal of Experimental Biology* 214, no.
2 (2011): 242–53. https://doi.org/10.1242/jeb.050989.

131 Gerald Keil, Elizabeth Cummings, and João Pedro de
Magalhães. "Being Cool: How Body Temperature Influences
Ageing and Longevity." *Biogerontology* 16, no. 4 (2015):
383–97. https://doi.org/10.1007/s10522-015-9571-2.

132 Jackson J. Fyfe, James R. Broatch, Adam J. Trewin, Erik D. Hanson, Christos K. Argus, Andrew P. Garnham, Shona L. Halson, Remco C. Polman, David J. Bishop, and Aaron C. Petersen. "Cold Water Immersion Attenuates Anabolic Signaling and Skeletal Muscle Fiber Hypertrophy, but Not Strength Gain, Following Whole-Body Resistance Training." *Journal of Applied Physiology* 127, no. 5 (2019): 1403–18. https://doi.org/10.1152/japplphysiol.00127.2019.

133 Gandhi Yetish, Hillard Kaplan, Michael Gurven, Brian Wood, Herman Pontzer, Paul R. Manger, Charles Wilson, Ronald McGregor, and Jerome M. Siegel. "Natural Sleep and Its Seasonal Variations in Three Pre-Industrial Societies." *Current Biology* 25, no. 21 (2015): 2862–68. https://doi.org/10.1016/j.cub.2015.09.046.

134 Megumi Hatori, C. Gronfier, R. N. Van Gelder, P. S. Bernstein, J. Carreras, S. Panda S, F. Marks D. Sliney, C. E. Hunt, T. Hirota, T. Furukawa, and K. Tsubota. "Global Rise of Potential Health Hazards Caused by Blue Light-Induced Circadian Disruption in Modern Aging Societies." NPJ aging and mechanisms of disease. U.S. National Library of Medicine, n.d. https://pubmed.ncbi.nlm.nih.gov/28649427/.

135 Aiha. "French Agency Examines Health Effects of Exposure to Blue Light." The Synergist. AIHA, October 18, 2021. https://synergist.aiha.org/201908-health-effects-blue-light.

136 Arnold Wilkins, Jennifer Veitch, and Brad Lehman. "LED Lighting Flicker and Potential Health Concerns: IEEE Standard par1789 Update." *2010 IEEE Energy Conversion Congress and Exposition*, 2010. https://doi.org/10.1109/ecce.2010.5618050.

137 Craig DiLouie and Malcolm Thomas. "IES Publishes Position Statement on Effects of Exterior Lighting on Human Health." LightNOW, August 30, 2010. http://www.lightnowblog.com/2010/09/ies-publishes-position-state-ment-on-effects-of-exterior-lighting-on-human-health/.

138 Joshua W. Mouland, Franck Martial, Alex Watson, Robert J. Lucas, and Timothy M. Brown. "Cones Support Alignment to an Inconsistent World by Suppressing Mouse Circadian Responses to the Blue Colors Associated with Twilight." *Current Biology* 29, no. 24 (2019). https://doi.org/10.1016/j.cub.2019.10.028.

139 Lucas Freitas de Freitas and Michael R Hamblin. "Proposed Mechanisms of Photobiomodulation or Low-Level Light Therapy." *IEEE Journal of Selected Topics in Quantum Electronics* 22, no. 3 (2016): 348–64. https://doi.org/10.1109/jstqe.2016.2561201.

140 Michael R. Hamblin. "Mechanisms and Applications of the Anti-Inflammatory Effects of Photobiomodulation." *AIMS Biophysics* 4, no. 3 (2017): 337–61. https://doi.org/10.3934/biophy.2017.3.337.

141 P. E. Watson, I. D. Watson, and R. D. Batt. "Total Body Water Volumes for Adult Males and Females Estimated from Simple Anthropometric Measurements." *The American Journal of Clinical Nutrition* 33, no. 1 (1980): 27–39. https://doi.org/10.1093/ajcn/33.1.27.

142 Ana Adan. "Cognitive Performance and Dehydration." *Journal of the American College of Nutrition* 31, no. 2 (2012): 71–78. https://doi.org/10.1080/07315724.2012.10720011.

143 Dietary Reference Intakes for Water, Potassium, Sodium, Chloride, and Sulfate" National Academies Press: OpenBook, n.d. https://www.nap.edu/read/10925/chapter/1.

144 Natalia I. Dmitrieva and Maurice B. Burg. "Elevated Sodium and Dehydration Stimulate Inflammatory Signaling in Endothelial Cells and Promote Atherosclerosis." *PLOS ONE* 10, no. 6 (2015). https://doi.org/10.1371/journal.pone.0128870.

145 Friedrich Manz and Andreas Wentz. "The Importance of Good Hydration for the Prevention of Chronic Diseases." *Nutrition Reviews* 63 (2005). https://doi.org/10.1111/j.1753-4887.2005.tb00150.x.

146 A. Kjaer, P. J. Larsen, U. Knigge, and J. Warberg. "Dehydration Stimulates Hypothalamic Gene Expression of Histamine Synthesis Enzyme: Importance for Neuroendocrine Regulation of Vasopressin and Oxytocin Secretion." *Endocrinology* 136, no. 5 (1995): 2189–97. https://doi.org/10.1210/endo.136.5.7720668.

147 François Péronnet, Diane Mignault, Patrick du Souich, Sébastien Vergne, Laurent Le Bellego, Liliana Jimenez, and Rémi Rabasa-Lhoret. "Pharmacokinetic Analysis of Absorption, Distribution and Disappearance of Ingested Water Labeled with D2O in Humans." *European Journal of Applied Physiology* 112, no. 6 (2011): 2213–22. https://doi.org/10.1007/s00421-011-2194-7.

148 Michael J. McKinley and Alan Kim Johnson. "The Physiological Regulation of Thirst and Fluid Intake." *Physiology* 19, no. 1 (2004): 1–6. https://doi.org/10.1152/nips.01470.2003.

149 Anna L. Choi, Guifan Sun, Ying Zhang, and Philippe Grandjean. "Developmental Fluoride Neurotoxicity: A Systematic Review and Meta-Analysis." *Environmental Health Perspectives* 120, no. 10 (2012): 1362–68. https://doi.org/10.1289/ehp.1104912.

150 Ryan Felton. "What's Really in Your Bottled Water?" Consumer Reports, September 24, 2020. https://www.consumerreports.org/water-quality/whats-really-in-your-bottled-water-a5361150329/.

151 Rafael de Cabo and Mark P. Mattson. "Effects of Intermittent Fasting on Health, Aging, and Disease." *New England Journal of Medicine* 381, no. 26 (2019): 2541–51. https://doi.org/10.1056/nejmra1905136.

152 M. Mattson and R. Wan. "Beneficial Effects of Intermittent Fasting and Caloric Restriction on the Cardiovascular and Cerebrovascular Systems." *The Journal of Nutritional Biochemistry* 16, no. 3 (2005): 129–37. https://doi.org/10.1016/j.jnutbio.2004.12.007.

153 Hiroshi Sogawa and Chiharu Kubo. "Influence of Short-Term Repeated Fasting on the Longevity of Female (NZB×NZW) F1 Mice." *Mechanisms of Ageing and Development* 115, no. 1-2 (2000): 61–71. https://doi.org/10.1016/s0047-6374(00)00109-3.

154 Yueming Zhu, Yufan Yan, David R. Gius, and Athanassios Vassilopoulos. "Metabolic Regulation of Sirtuins upon Fasting and the Implication for Cancer." *Current Opinion in Oncology* 25, no. 6 (2013): 630–36. https://doi.org/10.1097/01.cco.0000432527.49984.a3.

155 Leading Scientist in the Field of Nutrition." Dr. Paul Clayton, n.d. http://www.drpaulclayton.eu/.

156 Shao-Ming Wang, Jin-Hu Fan, Philip R. Taylor, Tram Kim Lam, Sanford M. Dawsey, You-Lin Qiao, and Christian C. Abnet. "Association of Plasma Vitamin C Concentration to Total and Cause-Specific Mortality: A 16-Year Prospective Study in China." *Journal of Epidemiology and Community Health* 72, no. 12 (2018): 1076–82. https://doi.org/10.1136/jech-2018-210809.

157 Olivier Bourron and Franck Phan. "Vitamin K." *Current Opinion in Clinical Nutrition & Metabolic Care* 22, no. 2 (2019): 174–81. https://doi.org/10.1097/mco.0000000000000541.

158 "What We Eat in America, NHANES 2005-2006 - USDA ARS," n.d. https://www.ars.usda.gov/ARSUserFiles/80400530/ pdf/0506/Table_1_NIN_GEN_05.pdf.

159 Bart A. Eijkelkamp, Jacqueline R. Morey, Stephanie L. Neville, Aimee Tan, Victoria G. Pederick, Nerida Cole, Prashina P. Singh, et al. "Dietary Zinc and the Control of Streptococcus Pneumoniae Infection." *PLOS Pathogens* 15, no. 8 (2019). https://doi.org/10.1371/journal.ppat.1007957.

160 Michalann Harthill. "Review: Micronutrient Selenium Deficiency Influences Evolution of Some Viral Infectious Diseases." *Biological Trace Element Research* 143, no. 3 (2011): 1325–36. https://doi.org/10.1007/s12011-011-8977-1.

161 Frank J. Wolters, Hazel I. Zonneveld, Silvan Licher, Lotte G. M. Cremers, M. Kamran Ikram, Peter J. Koudstaal, Meike W. Vernooij, and M. Arfan Ikram. "Hemoglobin and Anemia in Relation to Dementia Risk and Accompanying Changes on Brain MRI." *Neurology* 93, no. 9 (2019). https://doi.org/10.1212/wnl.0000000000008003.

162 Fulya Bakilan, Onur Armagan, Merih Ozgen, Funda Tascioglu, Ozge Bolluk, and Ozkan Alatas. "Effects of Native Type II Collagen Treatment on Knee Osteoarthritis: A Randomized Controlled Trial." *The Eurasian Journal of Medicine* 48, no. 2 (2016): 95–101. https://doi.org/10.5152/eurasianjmed.2015.15030.

163 Juybari K. Bahrampour, Mohammad Hossein Pourhanifeh, Azam Hosseinzadeh, Karim Hemati, and Saeed Mehrzadi. "Melatonin Potentials against Viral Infections Including COVID-19: Current Evidence and New Findings." *Virus Research* 287 (2020): 198108. https://doi.org/10.1016/j.virusres.2020.198108.

164 Meharban Singh. "Essential Fatty Acids, DHA and Human Brain." *The Indian Journal of Pediatrics* 72, no. 3 (2005): 239–42. https://doi.org/10.1007/bf02859265.

165 M. Elizabeth Sublette, Steven P. Ellis, Amy L. Geant, and J. John Mann. "Meta-Analysis of the Effects of Eicosapentaenoic Acid (EPA) in Clinical Trials in Depression." *The Journal of Clinical Psychiatry* 72, no. 12 (2011): 1577–84. https://doi.org/10.4088/jcp.10m06634.

166 Raffaele De Caterina, Rosalinda Madonna, and Marika Massaro. "Effects of Omega-3 Fatty Acids on Cytokines and Adhesion Molecules." *Current Atherosclerosis Reports* 6, no. 6 (2004): 485–91. https://doi.org/10.1007/s11883-004-0090-x.

167 A. P. Simopoulos. "The Importance of the Ratio of Omega-6/Omega-3 Essential Fatty Acids." *Biomedicine & Pharmacotherapy* 56, no. 8 (2002): 365–79. https://doi.org/10.1016/s0753-3322(02)00253-6.

168 Kirsty Brown, Daniella DeCoffe, Erin Molcan, and Deanna L. Gibson. "Diet-Induced Dysbiosis of the Intestinal Microbiota and the Effects on Immunity and Disease." *Nutrients* 4, no. 8 (2012): 1095–1119. https://doi.org/10.3390/nu4081095.

169 M. J. Butel. "Probiotics, Gut Microbiota and Health." *Médecine et Maladies Infectieuses* 44, no. 1 (2014): 1–8. https://doi.org/10.1016/j.medmal.2013.10.002.

170 Zhenchan Lu, Bi Rong Dong, Chang Quan Huang, and Taixiang Wu. "Probiotics for Preventing Acute Upper Respiratory Tract Infections." *Cochrane Database of Systematic Reviews*, 2008. https://doi.org/10.1002/14651858.cd006895.

171 L. Lehtoranta, A. Pitkäranta, and R. Korpela. "Probiotics in Respiratory Virus Infections." *European Journal of Clinical Microbiology & Infectious Diseases* 33, no. 8 (2014): 1289–1302. https://doi.org/10.1007/s10096-014-2086-y.

172 Giorgio La Fata, Robert Rastall, Christophe Lacroix, Hermie Harmsen, M. Mohajeri, Peter Weber, and Robert Steinert. "Recent Development of Prebiotic Research—Statement from an Expert Workshop." *Nutrients* 9, no. 12 (2017): 1376. https://doi.org/10.3390/nu9121376.

173 K. Tsilingiri and M. Rescigno. "Postbiotics: What Else?" *Beneficial Microbes* 4, no. 1 (2013): 101–7. https://doi.org/10.3920/bm2012.0046.

174 Eric Pelfrene, Elsa Willebrand, Ana Cavaleiro Sanches, Zigmars Sebris, and Marco Cavaleri. "Bacteriophage Therapy: A Regulatory Perspective." *Journal of Antimicrobial Chemotherapy* 71, no. 8 (2016): 2071–74. https://doi.org/10.1093/jac/dkw083.

175 Mehdi Jafari, Seyed Masood Mousavi, Asra Asgharzadeh, and Neda Yazdani. "Coenzyme Q10 in the Treatment of Heart Failure:

A Systematic Review of Systematic Reviews." *Indian Heart Journal* 70 (2018). https://doi.org/10.1016/j.ihj.2018.01.031.

176 R. Deichmann, C. Lavie, and S. Andrews. "Coenzyme Q10 and Statin-Induced Mitochondrial Dysfunction." The Ochsner journal. U.S. National Library of Medicine, n.d. https://pubmed.ncbi.nlm.nih.gov/21603349/.

177 Kyosuke Watanabe, Satoshi Nozaki, Miki Goto, Ken-ichi Kaneko, Emi Hayashinaka, Satsuki Irie, Akira Nishiyama, et al. "PET Imaging of 11C-Labeled Coenzyme Q10: Comparison of Biodistribution between [11c]Ubiquinol-10 and [11c]Ubiquinone-10." *Biochemical and Biophysical Research Communications* 512, no. 3 (2019): 611–15. https://doi.org/10.1016/j.bbrc.2019.03.073.

178 Renu Yadav, Babban Jee, and Sudhir Kumar Awasthi. "Curcumin Suppresses the Production of pro-Inflammatory Cytokine Interleukin-18 in Lipopolysaccharide Stimulated Murine Macrophage-like Cells." *Indian Journal of Clinical Biochemistry* 30, no. 1 (2014): 109–12. https://doi.org/10.1007/s12291-014-0452-2.

179 Giovanna Bianchi, Silvia Ravera, Chiara Traverso, Adriana Amaro, Francesca Piaggio, Laura Emionite, Tiziana Bachetti, Ulrich Pfeffer, and Lizzia Raffaghello. "Curcumin Induces a Fatal Energetic Impairment in Tumor Cells in Vitro and in Vivo by Inhibiting ATP-Synthase Activity." *Carcinogenesis* 39, no. 9 (2018): 1141–50. https://doi.org/10.1093/carcin/bgy076.

180 Albino Carrizzo, Maurizio Forte, Antonio Damato, Valentina Trimarco, Francesco Salzano, Michelangelo Bartolo, Anna Maciag, Annibale A. Puca, and Carmine Vecchione. "Antioxidant Effects of Resveratrol in Cardiovascular, Cerebral and Metabolic Diseases." *Food and Chemical Toxicology* 61 (2013): 215–26. https://doi.org/10.1016/j.fct.2013.07.021.

181 Troy L. Merry and Michael Ristow. "Do Antioxidant Supplements Interfere with Skeletal Muscle Adaptation to Exercise Training?" *The Journal of Physiology* 594, no. 18 (2016): 5135–47. https://doi.org/10.1113/jp270654.

182 Stephen E. Alway, Jean L. McCrory, Kalen Kearcher, Austen Vickers, Benjamin Frear, Diana L. Gilleland, Daniel E. Bonner,

et al. "Resveratrol Enhances Exercise-Induced Cellular and Functional Adaptations of Skeletal Muscle in Older Men and Women." *The Journals of Gerontology: Series A* 72, no. 12 (2017): 1595–1606. https://doi.org/10.1093/gerona/glx089.

183 Yusuf Abba, Hasliza Hassim, Hazilawati Hamzah, and Mohamed Mustapha Noordin. "Antiviral Activity of Resveratrol against Human and Animal Viruses." *Advances in Virology* 2015 (2015): 1–7. https://doi.org/10.1155/2015/184241.

184 Michael R. Lieber. "The Mechanism of Double-Strand DNA Break Repair by the Nonhomologous DNA End-Joining Pathway." *Annual Review of Biochemistry* 79, no. 1 (2010): 181–211. https://doi.org/10.1146/annurev.biochem.052308.093131.

185 Emre Koyuncu, Hanna G. Budayeva, Yana V. Miteva, Dante P. Ricci, Thomas J. Silhavy, Thomas Shenk, and Ileana M. Cristea. "Sirtuins Are Evolutionarily Conserved Viral Restriction Factors." *mBio* 5, no. 6 (2014). https://doi.org/10.1128/mbio.02249-14.

186 Andrew Blix. "Personalized Medicine, Genomics, and Pharmacogenomics." *Clinical Journal of Oncology Nursing* 18, no. 4 (2014): 437–41. https://doi.org/10.1188/14.cjon.437-441.

187 Gabor Marth, Raymond Yeh, Matthew Minton, Rachel Donaldson, Qun Li, Shenghui Duan, Ruth Davenport, Raymond D. Miller, and Pui-Yan Kwok. "Single-Nucleotide Polymorphisms in the Public Domain: How Useful Are They?" *Nature Genetics* 27, no. 4 (2001): 371–72. https://doi.org/10.1038/86864.

188 Stephany Tandy-Connor, Jenna Guiltinan, Kate Krempely, Holly LaDuca, Patrick Reineke, Stephanie Gutierrez, Phillip Gray, and Brigette Tippin Davis. "False-Positive Results Released by Direct-to-Consumer Genetic Tests Highlight the Importance of Clinical Confirmation Testing for Appropriate Patient Care." *Genetics in Medicine* 20, no. 12 (2018): 1515–21. https://doi.org/10.1038/gim.2018.38.

189 G. Bhanuprakash Reddy, V. Sudhakar Reddy, Ravindranadh Palika, Ayesha Ismail, and Raghu Pullakhandam. "Nutrigenomics: Opportunities & Challenges for Public Health Nutrition." *Indian Journal of Medical Research* 148, no. 5 (2018): 632. https://doi.org/10.4103/ijmr.ijmr_1738_18.

190 Lyle Armstrong. *Epigenetics*. New York, NY: Garland Science, 2014.

191 Elaine Schmidt. "Epigenetic Clock." Epigenetic Clock | Harvard Medical School, September 29, 2016. https://hms.harvard.edu/news/epigenetic-clock.

192 Martin Brunel Whyte and Philip Kelly. "The Normal Range: It Is Not Normal and It Is Not a Range." *Postgraduate Medical Journal* 94, no. 1117 (2018): 613–16. https://doi.org/10.1136/postgradmedj-2018-135983.

193 Ōura Partners with WNBA for 2020 Season." Business Wire, July 30, 2020. https://www.businesswire.com/news/home/20200730005532/en/%C2%A0Oura-Partners-With-WNBA-for-2020-Season.

194 Julia Belluz, Brad Plumer, and Brian Resnick. "The 7 Biggest Problems Facing Science, According to 270 Scientists." Vox. Vox, July 14, 2016. https://www.vox.com/2016/7/14/12016710/science-challeges-research-funding-peer-review-process.

195 Milton Packer. "What Freddie Mercury Can Teach Us About Clinical Trials." Medical News. MedpageToday, February 20, 2019. https://www.medpagetoday.com/opinion/revolutionandrevelation/78118.

196 Pathma D. Joseph, Jonathan C. Craig, and Patrina H.Y. Caldwell. "Clinical Trials in Children." *British Journal of Clinical Pharmacology* 79, no. 3 (2015): 357–69. https://doi.org/10.1111/bcp.12305.

197 Dr. Ananya Mandal, MD, "What is Autophagy?" Medical News, June 5, 2019, https://www.news-medical.net/life-sciences/What-is-Autophagy.aspx.

198 Robert K. Naviaux. "Metabolic Features of the Cell Danger Response." *Mitochondrion* 16 (2014): 7–17. https://doi.org/10.1016/j.mito.2013.08.006.

ACKNOWLEDGMENTS

I WANT TO ACKNOWLEDGE THE worst pandemic in a century. I extend compassion to those who lost loved ones but have to recognize that had I not been forced to cancel my schedule and remain at home for such a prolonged period of time, I would never have been able to sit still long enough to write this book.

This endeavor turned out to be one of the most intellectually engaging projects of my life.

I want to express my appreciation to the team at Post Hill Press, with particular thanks to Debra Englander for taking a chance on me and my manuscript. Her continued advice was valuable, and she was able to persuade me that my original 400-page manuscript was way too long. Thank you, Heather King, for guiding me through the process of publishing—a process I knew exactly nothing about. Thank you Herb Schaffner for all of your help.

Thank you to my wonderful sons who inspire me daily. I appreciate your unwavering patience with my constant technology mishaps. I love you both more than I can express and enjoy every precious moment that we spend together. Thank you, Mark, for feeding me and keeping me sane (although he insists the sanity part is debatable!). Thank you to my mother who I am pretty sure will buy a few books. Thank you, Larry Hite, for your guidance, mentoring, and excellent advice. Thank you, Bill Stanford, for encouraging me to write this book and continuing to represent the consumer perspective. I appreciate all of our conversations about Biology and Physiology. Thank you, Tim Shaheen, for your bravery in reading one of my unedited, long versions of my manuscript. Thank you, Nicole Yorkin, for all your suggestions and referrals That is a true friend! Thank you, Brett Johnson, for your constant encouragement and unbridled enthusiasm. Thank you, Chris Desser, for your terrific suggestions. Thank you, Carli Greenebaum and Victoria Filice, for always being there and our many conversations—often about nothing in particular.